Peter Mandel

# Acu-Impulsor Therapy

Treatment
With Piezoelectric Impulses

PETER MANDEL

# ACU-IMPULSOR THERAPY

## TREATMENT WITH PIEZOELECTRIC IMPULSES

EDITION ENERGETIK

Translated into English by Christopher Baker and Judith Harrison

| | |
|---|---|
| Cover | Rosita Reger |
| Layout | Siegfried Janusch |
| Photography | Fritsche & Wortmann, Mühlheim |
| Editor | Manfred Maiworm |
| Typesetting | Satzstudio K.H. Schumacher, Freiburg |
| Print | Freiburger Graphische Betriebe |

Printed in West Germany
ISBN 3-925806-11-3

Two years after the publication of the "Compendium of Colorpuncture" we are finally able to present "Acu-Impulsor Therapy".

I know that many people who have already been using the acu-impulsor PM 2001 for a considerable time have been awaiting the publication of this book with some impatience. I hope the reader will understand that my busy practice and the ongoing research work have left me with very little time to devote myself to providing the necessary medical literature, however important this may be. I am sure that the reader will appreciate that no efforts have been spared in the production of this book, which will hopefully prove its worth as a basic reference work for the effective use of the PM 2001 acu-impulsor.

"Acu-Impulsor Therapy" has been written for medical practitioners and the lay person alike. Those professionals employing energy oriented therapeutic methods in their practice may regard certain sections as being superfluous. Please bear in mind that acu-impulsor therapy is now being employed as a health preserving, health promoting self-help method by such a large number of lay persons that I felt it necessary to give all readers the opportunity to gain a beter understanding of how this form of therapy works.

I would like to impress upon the lay reader the fact that a thorough diagnosis by a physician or licensed health practitioner should always precede self-treatment.

Recently I have often been asked to explain the difference between acu-impulsor therapy and Colorpuncture and as to whether it is necessary to employ both methods and also if it would not suffice to opt for one or the other.

The answer is simple if one considers the different type of action the two methods exert on the energetic system.

Acu-impulsor therapy serves the purpose of regulating energy and is a fast-acting, energy-directing type of treatment. The impulse exerts an influence on the energy quality in terms of intensity and pace of flow. This is capable of overcoming energetic blockages and restoring the flow of information.

Colorpuncture acts on a higher energetic level and serves the purpose of regulating information. Colored light contains information which is "understood" by the cells, as it has been shown that the latter possess inherent light and color properties of their own. Colorpuncture is capable of reharmonizing disordered informational patterns.

Thus both methods have their own special significance and employment.

Acu-impulsor therapy is particularly suited for prophylactic use and the treatment of less severe conditions caused by disturbances of the energy flow.

Peter Mandel

# Introduction

The days of our unconditional faith in progress are over. As individuals, we are forced to look at other, less fortuitous facets of our highly technological world, as exemplified by accumulating catastrophes; and realize the dangers involved.

The more obvious it becomes that man is divesting himself of his own natural conditions for life, the greater becomes the wish in many people to return to a state of harmony with nature.
Particularly in the field of health care, this trend is unmistakable. With medicine becoming increasingly technical, sickness being reduced to purely physical symptoms and the amount of frightening information on the damaging side effects of many kinds of medicine, more and more people are turning back to natural methods of healing.

Apart from licensed health practitioners, an increasing number of doctors are turning to natural healing methods, although they do not always meet with praise among their colleagues. The advantage of natural healing methods is that therapy is not confined to bombarding the symptoms of a disease process with the heaviest artillery available; instead, attention is paid to uncovering the hidden causes. On the basis of his whole philosophy of life, the practitioner of natural therapeutics regards disease as the physical expression of a disturbance in the complex overall system of the person involved. Acknowledgement of the metaphysical threefold nature of human existence, as reflected in the interaction of body, mind and spirit, means that it is necessary to include several levels of interpretation in the search for root causes.

Natural therapeutics consist of a number of theories and methods, of which most, however, have a common denominator. They define the true sustainer of life as a vital energy. They claim that this central force is responsible for all life processes. Sickness and disease are viewed as an energetic imbalance in the overall system, and therapeutic measures are aimed at reharmonizing this imbalance in the flow of energy.

In view of this, it is hardly surprising that, since coming into contact with natural therapeutics, I have devoted myself to research into the nature of this life energy. Such happy circumstances as the discovery of Kirlian photography by the Soviet scientist of the same name, and my own scientific interest in finding out more about the phenomenon of "bioenergy" enabled me, with the help of acupuncture and other new methods of diagnosis and therapy, to develop Energy Emission Analysis (EEA) and Colorpuncture, both of which are based entirely on the knowledge and principles of energy. My methods indicate a connection between the apparently incompatible. However, without thousands of years of traditional Chinese medicine, progress in high frequency photography and the development of a Colorpuncture apparatus with its glass fiber light conductors, these new methods would have been inconceivable.

I have therefore come to the conclusion that modern technology is a means whereby we can render more transparent the secrets of life, the complexity of which man has always sensed. What is surprising is that so-called modern scientific findings are frequently no more than a confirmation of the deep knowledge that has been traditionally passed on from one generation to another and which even today is often dismissed as quackery.

The excellent results that can be achieved with these methods have attracted people from all over the Federal Republic of Germany and abroad to my practice in Bruchsal.

Many of these patients are prepared to journey hundreds of kilometers. The inconvenience involved, both in terms of time and money, gave rise to the very understandable wish for a system which could be applied at home and which would stabilize the success of treatment carried out in my practice.

As long as this only involved concomitant medication, it was no problem meeting this wish. But how could I continue to help those who had been treated with acupuncture or who had received treatment in the form of injection into acupuncture points?

Challenged in this way, I set out to find a therapy form which:

a) is based on my methods

b) can be practiced by the layperson

c) fulfills my demands in terms of efficacy, which are certainly not negligible.

Since, as has already been stated, my therapeutic ideas presuppose the existence of a life energy which controls all life processes, it was logical to search for "something" which would exert a similar influence on the overall balance of energy, as can be achieved, for instance, through acupuncture with needles.

In the course of my research studies and discussions carried out with many colleagues, it occurred to me that the piezoelectric effect might contribute to the solution of this problem. This effect, which occurs in quartz watches, lighters, etc., stems from the property of certain crystals, e.g. quartz, to develop electrical surface tension when placed under pressure. Given an appropriate construction, this electric tension discharges in the form of sparks, and to my mind there had to be some way of channelling this tension into the overall energetic system via the acupuncture points.

I then had Vega, a firm in Schiltach, West Germany, develop the so-called acu-impulsor. Its use in practice confirms daily that I had been thinking along the right lines: when applied to the respective acupuncture points, the piezoelectric charge triggers off an initial impulse which reproduces itself in a wavelike movement within the energetic system, balancing out and harmonizing discordant energetic vibrations in the process.

In order to gain a better understanding of the acu-impulsor, I consider it necessary to give a summary of Chinese acupuncture in the following chapter.

# Acupuncture

It is futile to attempt to fathom out the beginnings of the traditional Chinese healing method of acupuncture. It is, however, known that it has been practiced for many thousands of years and that it was first expressed in writing some 600 years B.C. The theory is based on the idea that the human body contains a dense network of invisible channels through which "chi", the fundamental life force, flows. This "chi" is, however, not merely a Chinese concept. Almost all cultures, including those of ancient Egypt, India, Greece and Rome, have believed in this life-giving energy. In the metaphysics and mysteries of the Gnostic, Neoplatonic, Jewish and ancient Christian traditions, in the secret Hermetic teachings and in alchemy, in Renaissance medicine and in Humanism, chi has always been a factor of central importance, whatever the name it was given.

In all languages, people have always given what we call the soul names which stand for an almost imperceptible form of materiality, names like waft and wind, or breath or zephyr. These images are borrowed from the natural process of transpiration. The realization that life is inseparably bound to breathing and that without breathing, the body would become a corpse, led to the recognition that *psyche* (breath) and *los* (life) are identical. Clearly, the people of long ago found it easier to handle the mysteries of life in a concrete, rational way. They expressed this in an almost mathematical manner: the difference between a body and a corpse is life; therefore, the sustainer of life must be a mysterious form of energy.

The Chinese took it upon themselves to discover how this life energy circulates through the body. They found out that it does so in regular patterns and that it is present in all parts of the body at all times.

Over the millenia, it has been an incredibly painstaking task to find the network of channels through which chi flows. These channels, or meridians, which bear an amazing similarity to an irrigation system, connect all the different parts of the body and control and maintain the normal functioning of the bioorganism. Normal functioning, i.e. health, is maintained as long as chi is spread evenly and homogeneously throughout the system and can flow through the invisible web of meridians at its own pace and in a balanced manner. A person feels well and healthy if all the meridians are filled with an equal quantity of chi. If, however, it becomes congested or diminished in any region of the body, or if it stops flowing altogether in parts, a state of imbalance will occur. The under- or oversupplied meridians will be weakened and no longer able to resist pathogenic agents, i.e. disease-causing forces. Pathogenic agents also travel via the meridian system, which means that diseases of the inner organs, for instance, will be accompanied by symptoms on the surface of the body or in the extremities and joints. All acupuncturists formulate the phenomenon more or less in this way. Needles are applied to the points of the body where the meridians run close beneath the surface of the skin in order to reach and stimulate the meridian or meridians as a means of reharmonizing the quantity and rate of flow of chi. The main meridians run parallel to the vertical axis of the patient. There are twelve main channels and eight special ones, all interconnected via side channels, horizontal channels, bifurcations and ramifications and collectively forming a single circulatory system. Three of the twelve main meridians meet at their end points, which are to be found at the tips of the fingers, the end joints of the toes, in the head and in the chest. The three yin meridians of the hand, which start in the chest and end in the fingers (where they meet the three yang meridians of the hand, which begin in the tips of the fingers and end in the head), fuse in the tips of the toes with the three yin meridians of the foot. These last go from the feet to the chest, where they meet the three yin meridians of the hand. In addition to the main meridians already named, an ever-increasing number of so-called lesser meridians have been discovered in the course of time. The terms yin and yang are of paramount importance to Chinese philosophy and practical acupuncture. However, these two concepts did not originate in acupuncture, but have their roots in an all-embracing, religious view of the world. In Taoism, yin and yang symbolize interrelated polarities governing the whole of the cosmos, the course of time and all that is of this world, including the human individual and his bioorganism. The mystic, symbolic notion of polarity has been a feature of philosophy at all times. When attempting to define magneticism and electricity, the natural sciences were forced at the very latest to accept the fact that a description of these phenomena is impossible without taking the concept of polarity into consideration.

In contrast to widespread belief, the yin/yang polarity of Taoism by no means expresses a hierarchy of values. Yang as the male, positive pole stands as little for good in a moral sense as does yin, the female, negative pole, for evil. Both poles are equal in value, each conditions the other and each is dependent upon the presence of the opposite pole for its *raison d'être*. Yin represents the earth, femaleness, receptivity, softness, darkness, weakness, surrender and passivity. Yang is heaven, maleness, creativity, activity, procreation, hardness, resilience, aggression, lightness, warmth and strength.

This symbolism makes it clear that, in accordance with the Chinese view of things, only the equality of yin and yang can maintain the cosmos as it is and that all parts of this cosmos are subject to the same principles. Yin and yang always even out to a state of harmony, symmetry and balanced proportion, they retain equilibrium like the two sides of a set of scales. Whether in cybernetic feedback control systems, in the Gestalt theory in psychology or in the self-regulation of autonomous neurological systems, the polarity of yin and yang is always present but described in other terms.

According to Taoist philosophy, yin and yang dwell in Tao, as safe as a watch in its case. Tao forces them together into a ball or two-dimensional circle. Tao means way, path, direction. As far as the individual is concerned, Tao amounts to "being condemned to existence" as Sartre once put it, or the "state of being flung" (into existence) as Heidegger understood it. But Tao is also a good power, merciful and loving like God. Tao is all things within the cosmos, the irrevocable natural law to which one must submit without demur. More recent religions have called it by other names, such as Jahveh, Adar or God, describing a deity whose unfathomable decrees must be followed without contradiction, as must the mysterious rotation of Tao.

Theories regarding the microcosm and macrocosm, upper and lower, were not first developed by Western metaphysics. Long before that, the Chinese were convinced that the human being corresponds to Tao as the connecting link between heaven and earth and that the supreme forces of yin and yang determine man as a whole and the individual parts of his body. For this reason, the first and foremost concern of Chinese therapists is to ensure that the forces of yin and yang retain or achieve a state of balance within the body. Acupuncture is used as a means of prophylaxis in order to prevent the occurrence of acute disease, which can only emerge if a state of imbalance is allowed to linger. Ideally, a Chinese doctor need never treat manifest acute or chronic disease. He regards himself as the stimulator of the self-healing powers of the organism.

In the course of their very long history, Chinese Tao acupuncturists gradually discovered that by applying needles to a particular series of main points in succession, they could cause the symptoms of disease to disappear in a particular organ, which could thus be clearly attributed to these points. The early acupuncturists then joined these points, which were precisely marked on complicated diagrams, by an imaginary line. These lines later became the meridians. In the course of time they were able to attribute each meridian to a particular organ and determine the effect of applying the needles to each one of the innumerable acupuncture points. The application of this procedure can be traced back as far as about 2000 years BC. Evidence in writing and diagrams date back to about 500 BC. The earliest acupuncturists stimulated certain areas of the skin with sharpened, pointed stones; later they went on to use copper needles, then iron ones and, later still, silver and gold. The needles in use today are of a special steel alloy. The fact that the person treated was overcome by a sense of heaviness, relaxation and release of tension prompted the acupuncturists to seek new points in order to influence the state of the patient in a positive way. In the course of the dissemination of Chinese culture, the Japanese adopted the acupuncture technique in about 500 AD and developed it considerably. Today, we have access to documentation on acupuncture from countries with totally different political systems: China, Taiwan, Japan, Singapore and, in particular, France and Germany. This diversity of sources and the different methods currently in use ensures mutual control between the different schools of acupucture, meaning that if any kind of quackery occurrs, it will be forcefully denounced. However, this is by no means the only indication that the theory of acupuncture is correct. When acupuncture became known as a therapeutic method in the Western hemisphere, some 100 years ago, there was – understandably – great scepticism. There was no room within the basic philosophy of Western medicine, bound as it is to the constraints of exact scientific methods, for a healing system which is characterized by symbols, religious elements and objectively incorrect concepts. For instance, the ancient Chinese believed that the earth was a flat disc, and, as a consequence, they believed that heaven was above and the earth below. Those who, despite their scepticism, put the method to the test were therefore extremely astonished to find out how efficient treatment with acupuncture is. Acupuncture was then scrutinized for scientific substantiation of this phenomenon. Among other things, it was found that at the acupuncture points, the electric resistance and tension of the skin differed considerably from all other areas of the skin. It was thus possible to exactly determine the acupuncture points by measurement. The concept of chi presents greater difficulties because Western medicine still has no definition for life energy.

Even in China today, where Western medicine and acupuncture exist side by side, doctors now assume that acupuncture can only be applied to certain diseases and is not suitable in all cases. There is room for doubt as to whether this assumption is correct. Obviously, there is no substitute for modern intensive-care medicine. However, one is justified in asking whether intensive-care medicine would be necessary to the same degree if the basic philosophy behind acupuncture, namely that of maintaining the equilbrium of yin and yang, was firmly rooted in our consciousness and thus determined our actions. Anyone who regards acupuncture as antiquated and as a superfluous relict of days gone by can convince himself daily that this is not the case. Acupuncture is as alive as it ever was, for although man may not be able to define it, he can make use of it to manipulate his body – a fact which has always been, and will always be, absolutely fascinating.

From my point of view, it is important to point out that at no time was healing ever a materialistic, mechanic procedure. Man is not a machine in which worn-out parts can be replaced at will – even if there are many who would like to think so. Only when we come to understand that sickness is merely the expression of a disturbance within the overall energy system, will we realize that all areas of our being, including the mental and spiritual, are likewise affected. Consequently, all therapeutic measures must aim at healing man as a whole. They cannot be restricted to eliminating or – as occurs more frequently – suppressing physical symptoms.

This clearly demonstrates the advantage of energy-regulating forms of treatment: by influencing the flow of circulating energy and balancing out energetic disequilibrium, the person can be treated as a whole.

# The Use of the Acu-Impulsor

The previous chapter represented an introduction to an energetic, holistic approach as demonstrated by the theory of acupuncture.

The effect of the acu-impulsor can be conceived as follows: a piezoelectric charge is generated by pushing the button on the impulsor. This charge is channelled into the acupuncture point via a spark. The impulse thus triggered spreads out in waves along the respective meridian. A sluggish, reduced or blocked flow of energy is thus more or less pushed along until it regains its appropriate, harmonious rhythm. The regulative adjustment usually results in a rapid subjective and objective improvement of current ailments.

Many people who have no previous knowledge of acupuncture are puzzled by the fact that, for instance, in order to treat a headache, points are used in the foot or hand. One reason for this is that the acupuncture points, i.e. the points where the meridians run particularly close beneath the surface of the skin, are often situated far away from the region to be treated. The energetic information is transported from the acupuncture point via the meridians to the actual area affected by sickness.

The other, more important reason is that ailments are merely symptoms but not the cause of illness. A headache may have its root cause in disturbances in such areas as the urogenital tract, the stomach, the intestines or the psyche. It goes without saying that it is the cause that must be treated and not the symptoms. A headache can be eliminated, for instance, by treating the stomach.

Having explained the use and effect of the acu-impulsor, I shall now begin with instructions for the self-treatment of different ailments and diseases.

Natural therapeutics is an empirical science. It is based on experience gathered by natural healers throughout history. The importance and efficacy of acupuncture points, zones and segments as extraordinary therapeutic areas have repeatedly been proven in practice. For instance, pains in the knee, irrespective of their origin, may be connected to the lymphatic tonsillar ring and the tonsils; the cause of early morning backache is almost always rooted in intestinal problems. And women who suffer migraines before or after their periods can surely not be cured by being prescribed migraine remedies. One only has to think of the widespread occurence of mental disturbance, stress and depression. As a rule, the root causes are never taken into account. The list of diseases and ailments in which the causes are not identical to the symptoms is long and could be continued *ad infinitum.* Pain is nothing but a signal or – as a well-known German doctor put it – it is tissue crying out for the flow of energy. Assuming that this is the case, it is a prerequisite that the human energetic system should vibrate in a balanced rhythm. This is essential because life energy is the agent for vital information, which must flow harmoniously for every second of our lives. When it does not do so, the result is a disturbance in some part of our bodies. Disturbances and malfunctioning also form a source of information – they have the effect of an interfering transmitter. In this sense, the exchange of information is also subject to the laws of polarity. If feedback from the periphery is disturbed or distorted, the self-healing powers of the body will be immediately mobilized, but if the spread of false information cannot be prevented, disease will break out with all its symptoms. It is therefore imperative that we understand the coherency of the body in its entire complexity. We have to acknowledge that information is of paramount importance to our bodies and that the eternal circulation of flowing energy has no other function than to carry this information into all, even the minutest, areas of our life. All disturbances can be regulated when seen from this perspective, and a harmonious life, free of pain and burden, can be achieved by following the instructions set out in this book.

If done so in time, some "interfering transmitters" can be retuned to the right "frequency". However, this does not mean to say that this method of self-treatment can be seen as a panacea for all diseases and syndromes. On principle, all therapy must be preceded by a diagnosis. In the following I shall therefore distinguish between health-sustaining measures, which I call "energy balancing" and those destined to restore health. All ailments should first be diagnosed in order to ensure that serious, possibly concealed illnesses are not overlooked. It is necessary to know what is the matter before you start treatment and only a doctor or licensed health practitioner can make an accurate diagnosis, so consult one first of all. It is, of course, both legitimate and right to treat pain or so-called bagatelle ailments yourself or try to return the system to a state of peace, harmony and normal functioning with the help of medication. However, if the symptoms persist, you should go to a doctor or a licensed health practitioner.
By stimulating the congested or blocked energy potential, the piezoelectric impulse transmitted by the acu-impulsor can normalize the whole feedback control system. By treating yourself with the acu-impulsor, you balance your energy and help prevent disease and painful states. It is fundamentally important to allow yourself to be guided by the possible causes of a disease in order to approach bioenergetic processes in a holistic way. All the information in this book concerning the combinations of points and zone segments is based on years of experience with acupuncture and segmental and reflexotherapy.

Let us begin with energy balancing itself. This consists of:
1) general balancing of the energy flow,
2) strengthening of the immune system,
3) regulation of the control information.

# 1. General Balancing of the Energy Flow

In the mid-fifties, a physiotherapist by the name of Willi Penzel began to develop acupuncture massage. Today this is one of the few energy therapy methods which, when properly learnt, enables one to regulate the overall energy system of the body in an astonishingly simple way. Many practicing physiotherapists now use this beneficial method of treatment, which works by treating the meridian system. In his books, Willi Penzel describes the interaction of the human energy system in a simple and impressive way. During one of my Kirlian seminars in 1977 I had the opportunity of discussing energetic systems with this man. At the time we were both extremely pleased to find that our views on the matter corresponded to a high degree. He gave me *Energy Theory,* a booklet which he wrote with Dr. Reiners, and it still has its place on my desk today, albeit a little dog-eared. This translation of complicated Chinese works into a simple description of human energy systems has never ceased to fascinate me. I immediately incorporated many of the ideas on the meridian and the simple manipulations into my thoughts on treatment with the acu-impulsor. Penzel's basic assumption is that the meridians are similar to a system of canals in which the flow of water is controlled by means of weirs and locks. The first lock allows the water to flow in and the second canal lets it flow out. With regard to the meridians, this means that energy flows into the meridian at the first point and leave at the last. Within a canal system there are branches and a number of ditches which supply certain areas with water – in our case, with energy. The water level in these subsidiary canals is regulated by means of valves – the acupuncture points. All these valve-like acupuncture points have specific indications according to their value and are responsible for the abundance or lack of energy in their assigned regions. When treating with the acu-impulsor, attention is focussed on the first and last acupuncture points of a meridian. This alone does not constitute the cure for disease, but, on so-called healthy days, it can prevent sickness or at least alleviate minor ailments. Let us once again reflect on the fact that human life is subject to the universal laws of information and energy. Information which is peacefully transmitted through the meridian system within the energy potential can never cause disturbance in the overall system. However, in view of the conditions of modern life, such as environmental stress, false nutrition, etc., congestion and slight blockages in the flow of energy can occur frequently. Our self-healing powers, which might be likened to a repair crew that is permanently on the job, have their hands full simply maintaining the balance of yin and yang.

With the help of the acu-impulsor, we are in a position to prevent the strain on our energy potential from resulting in sickness. It is therefore suggested that you start with energy balancing, which consists of the three elements mentioned above. The first step is to treat the meridians as taught by Penzel. The first and last points of the meridians are stimulated with the acu-impulsor. My many years of experience with sick people have shown that by treating the twelve meridians in a certain way, one can eliminate many minor ailments. Attention must be paid to the connections between the meridians and maximum times of application. It takes only three x one minute per day to stimulate the meridians. Three minutes, which – if applied early enough – can bring lifelong reward. Even before disturbances manifest themselves within the flow of life energy, these three minutes will balance out your energy.

Different meridians are treated at different times of the day, with certain ones being treated in the morning, others at midday and others in the evening. The morning impulses apply to the meridians for the liver, gallbladder, colon and lungs. Always treat the first and last points of the meridians. The points come in pairs positioned on the left and right-hand side of the meridians. In all self-therapy with the acu-impulsor, always start on the left-hand side of the body.

For the sake of simplicity, I have numbered the points in question and put the names of the acupuncture points in brackets.

# General Balancing of the Energy Flow

Energy Balancing I
Energy Balancing II
Energy Balancing III

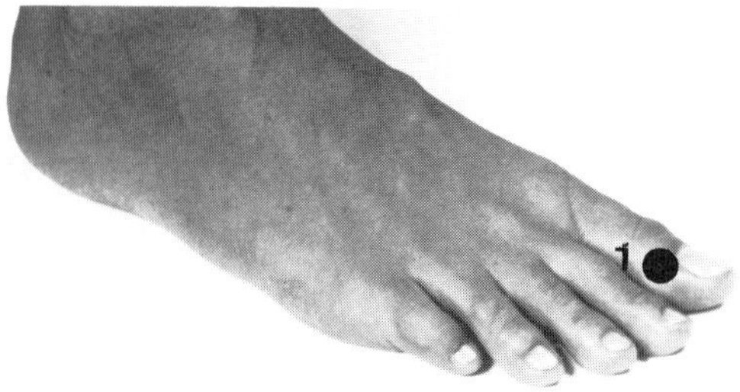


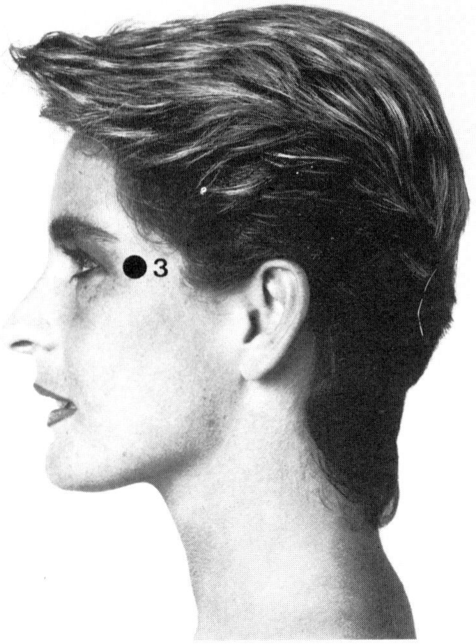


**Point 1**
(Liv. 1) Left and right
Located on the side facing 2nd toe, 2 mm at a diagonal from the angle of the nailbed.

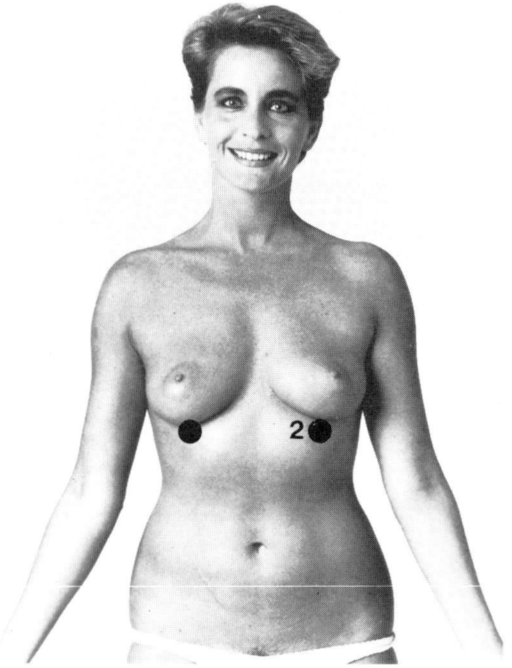


**Point 3**
(G.B. 1) Left and right
Located in the angle formed by the outer edge of the orbital arch and the cheek bone.

**Point 2**
(Liv. 14) Left and right
Located vertically beneath the nipple in the 5th intercostal space.

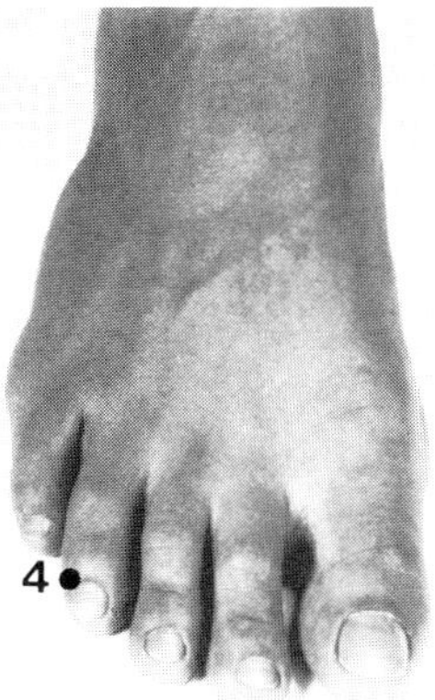


**Point 4**
(G.B. 44) Left and right
Located at the outer angle of the nailbed groove of the 4th toenail (facing the little toe), approx. 2 mm diagonally from the angle.

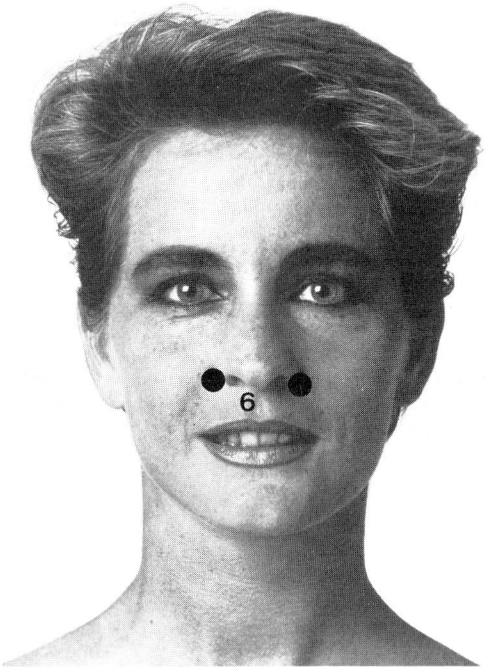


**Point 6**
(L.I. 20) Left and right
Located to the side of the nostril, a few millimeters from the nasolabial groove.

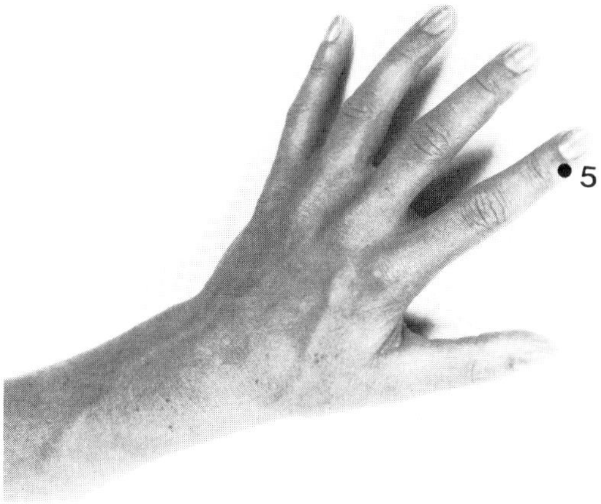


**Point 5**
(L.I. 1) Left and right
Located on the distal phalanx of the forefinger (thumb side), 2 mm diagonally away from the angle of the nail.

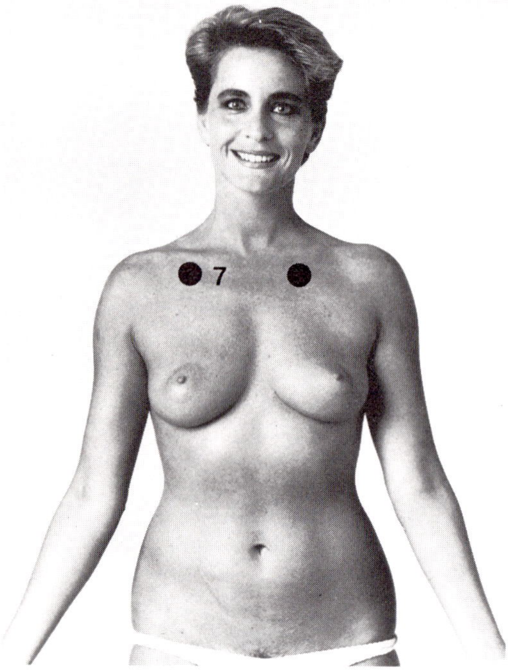


**Point 7:**
(Lu. 1) Left and right
Located a fingerbreadth from the lower edge of the collar-bone in the middle of the 1st intercostal space.

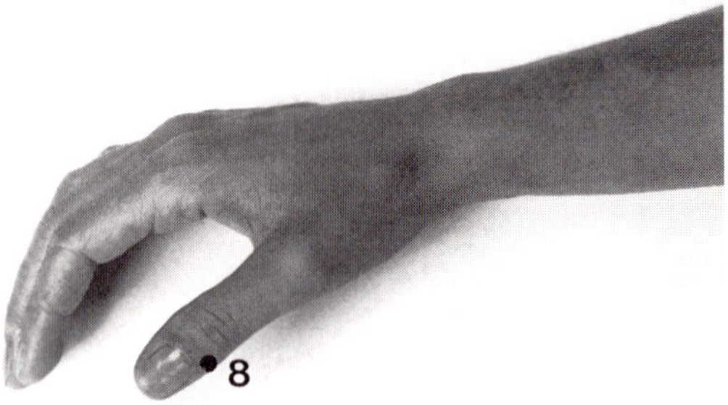


**Point 8:**
(Lu. 11) Left and right
Located on the lateral surface of the distal phalanx, 2 mm away from the angle of the nailbed.

Please use the illustrations as a guide and give each of these points ten impulses at one-second intervals.

The midday program includes the first and last points of the following meridians.

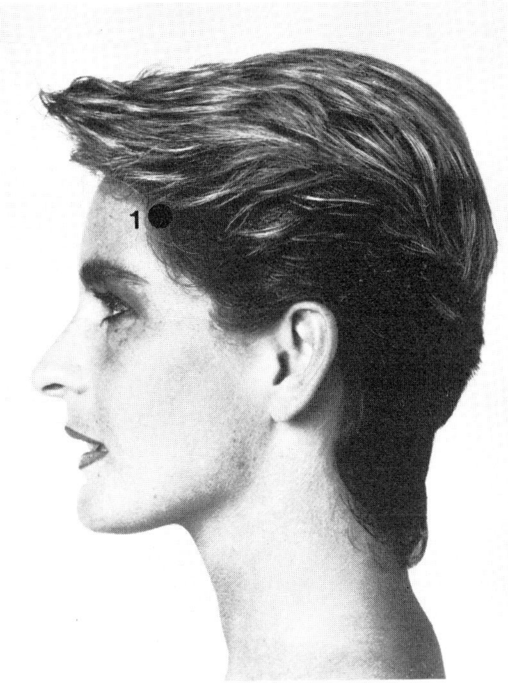


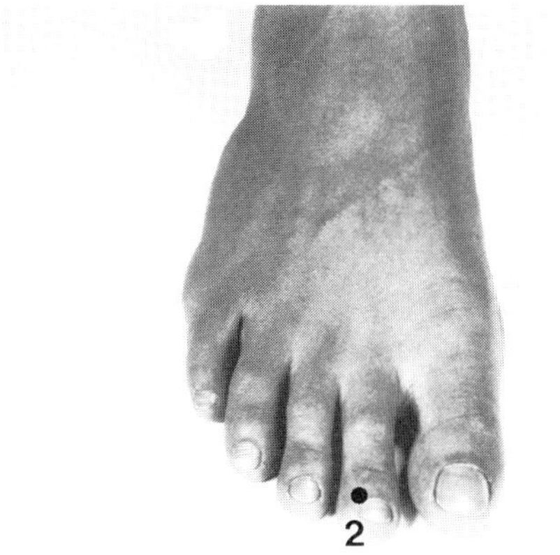


**Point 2**
(St. 45) Left and right
Located at the exterior corner of the 2nd toenail (pointing towards the little toe), about 2 mm diagonally from the angle of the nailbed.

**Point 1**
(St. 1) Left and right
Located in upper temple region, 4 fingerbreadths above and 1 fingerbreadth behind the orbital margin.

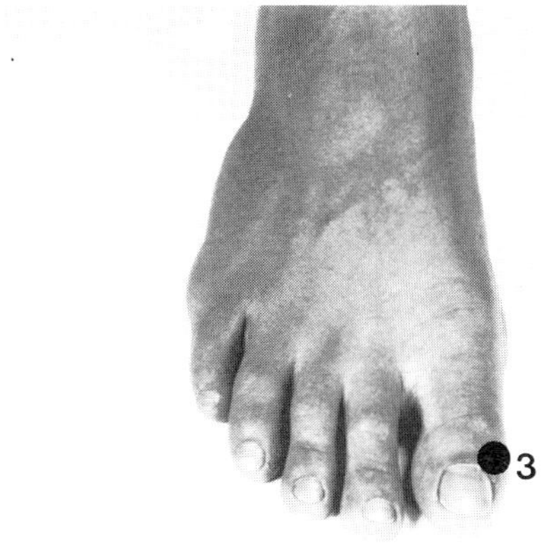


**Point 3**
(P. 1) Left and right
Located medially on the distal phalanx of the big toe, about 2 mm from the angle of the nailbed.

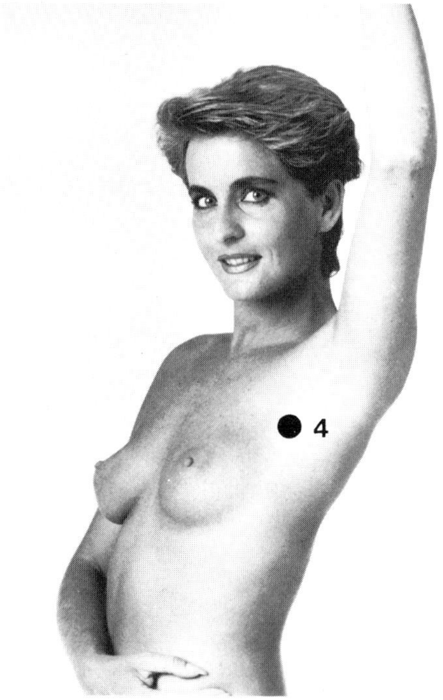


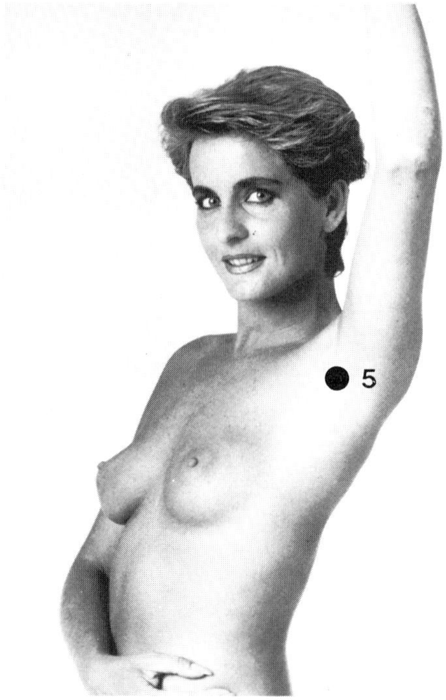


**Point 4**
(P. 21) Left and right
Located between the 6th intercostal space on the frontal axilliary line.

**Point 5**
(H. 1) Left and right
Located on lower edge of the third rib on the inner axilliary line.

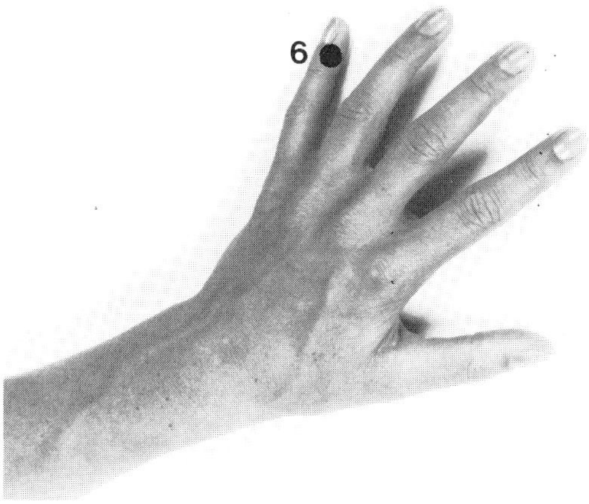


**Point 6**
(H. 9) Left and right
Located 2 mm from the medial angle of the nailbed on the little finger.

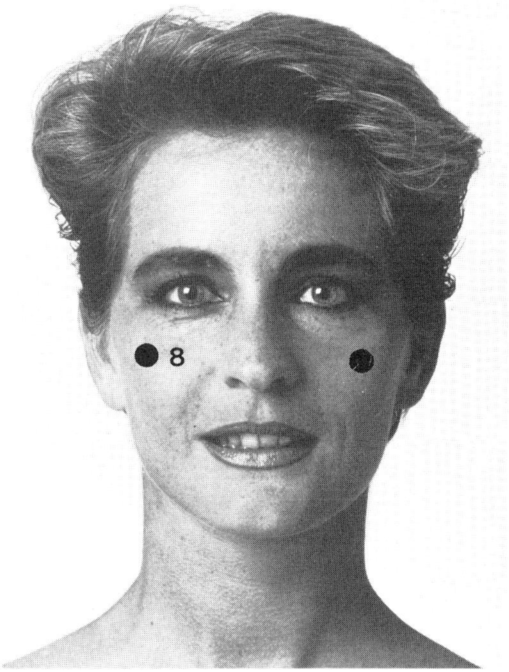


**Point 8**
(S.I. 18) Left and right
Located on the cheekbone beneath the outer corner of the eye where a small hollow can be felt.

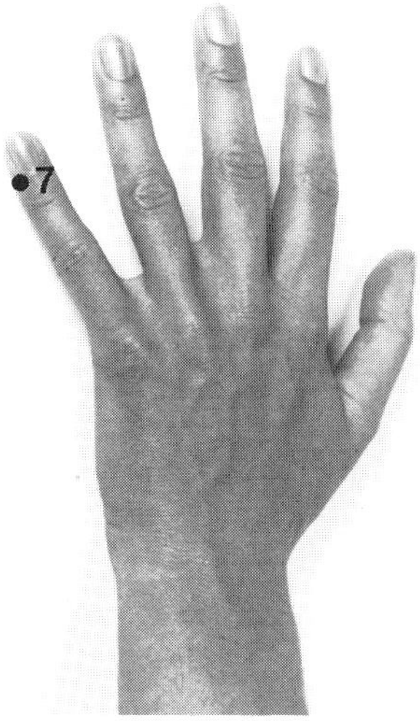


**Point 7**
(S.I. 1) Left and right
Located laterally on the distal phalanx of the little finger, 2 mm away from the lateral angle of the nailbed.

Here again, 10 impulses per pair of points should be applied, beginning on the left side.

The remaining meridians are stimulated in the evening, again with 10 impulses and beginning on the left side.

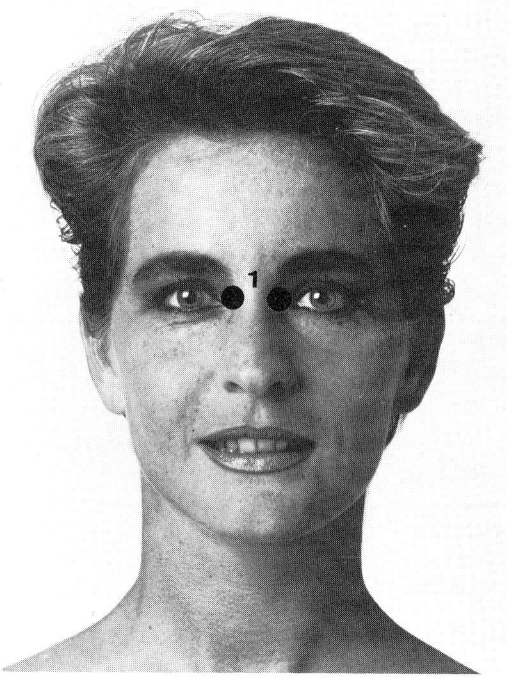


**Point 1**
(U.B. 1) Left and right
Located in the top inner corner of the eye socket.

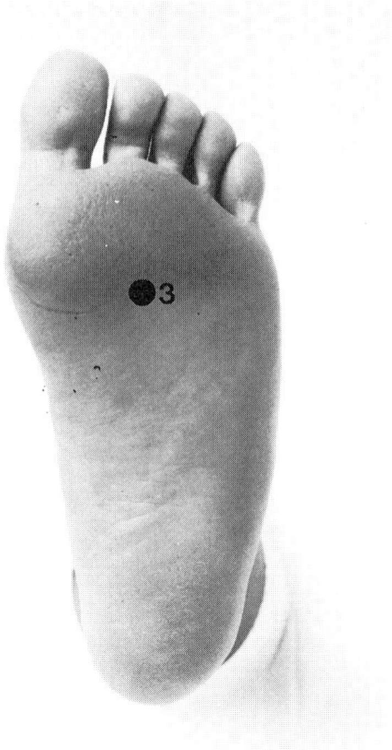


**Point 3**
(K. 1) Left and right
Located in the center of the ball of the foot.

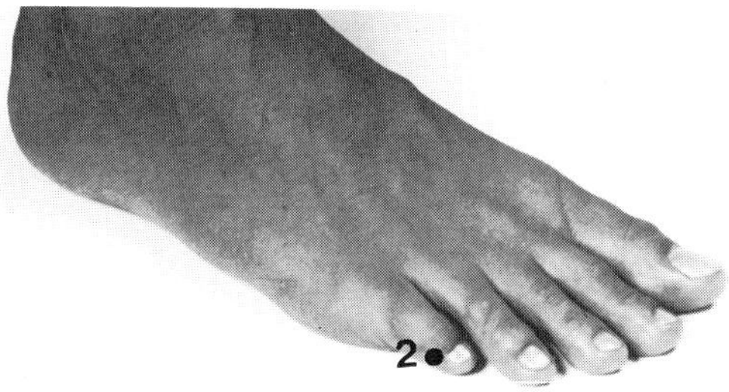


**Point 2**
(U.B. 67) Left and right
Located in the nailbed groove 2 mm away from the lateral angle of the nailbed on the little toe.

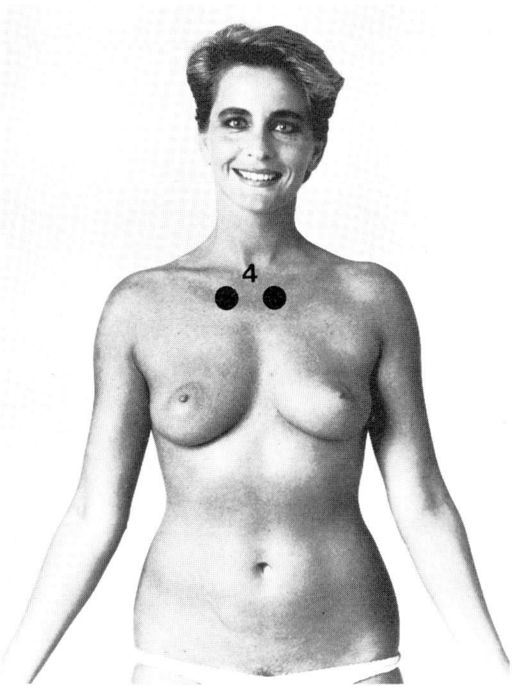


**Point 4**
(K. 27) Left and right
Located on the lower edge of the collar-bone, where it forms a joint with the breastbone

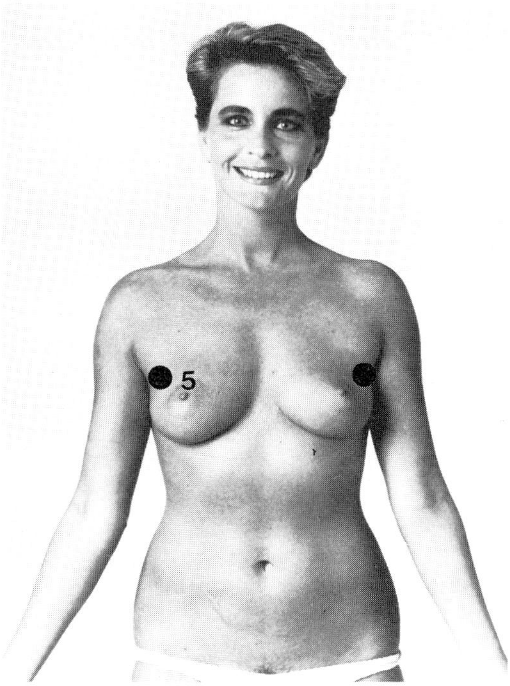


**Point 5**
(C. 1) Left and right
Located in the 4th intercostal space, 1 finger-breadth to the lateral side of the nipple.

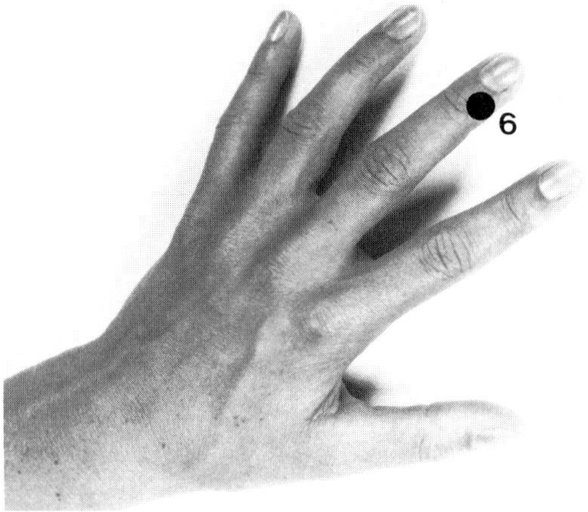


**Point 6**
(C. 9) Left and right
Located on the distal phalanx of the middle finger, 2 mm away from the angle of the nailbed groove.

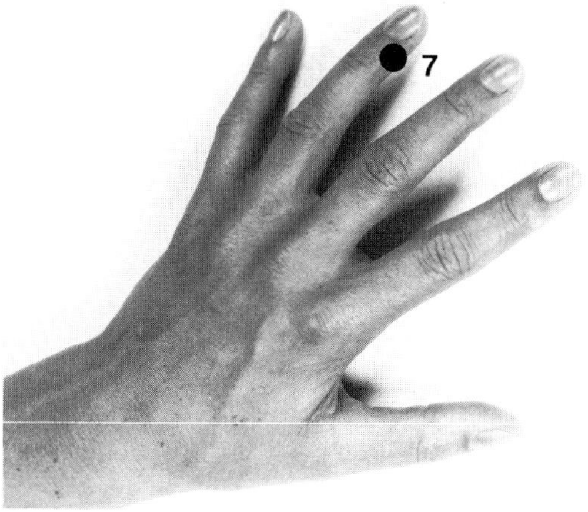


**Point 7**
(T.H. 1) Left and right
Located on the ring finger, 2 mm away from the lateral angle of the nailbed.

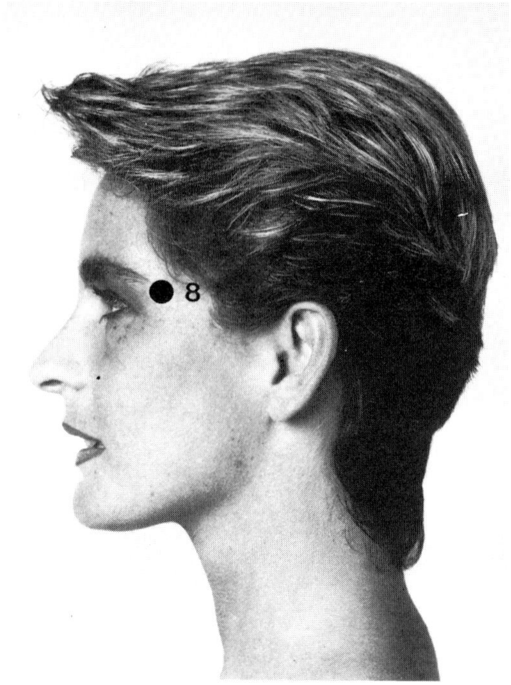


**Point 8**
(T.H. 23A) Left and right
Located at the outer end of the eyebrow.

Remember, only three minutes twice a week for a programm which can be extremely beneficial to you! Experience and observation have shown that this form of meridian treatment is truly an excellent way of balancing the body's energy.

# Strengthening the Immune System

It is only since AIDS has become an urgent issue that science has begun to pay greater attention to one of the most important systems in our bodies: the immune system, which can be compared with a batallion on permanent alert. However, the immune system is not any one organ, it is – like all systems – the sum of a multitude of functions; i.e. many cells, organs and other systems are involved in organising our body's defenses. These include the lymphatic system, which is so sadly overlooked in mainstream medicine. The lymphatic system is like a waste disposal unit and, according to the observations of natural therapists, fulfills an eminently important function within the immune system. My research into the Kirlian effect and the resultant method of Energy Emission Analysis (EEA) place the lymphatic system in the very foreground of energetic diagnosis. I have been able to discover, or rediscover, connections which allow a better understanding of the body's defense mechanisms. These are new zones and points independent of acupuncture; the resulting proposals for treatment are now being used successfully in many practices. The lymphatic system, therefore, has an important position within the body's functions.

As long as ten years ago, I worked out a combination of points which I was able to treat with piezoelectric impulses with great success. The following interconnected points have a preventive function, e.g. against colds, rheumatism, general weakness and for the detoxification of the organism. During the first 14 days of self-treatment, you should use the acu-impulsor to stimulate the organism as described below every morning. Ten impulses are to be given at one second intervals, starting on the left hand side of the body in each case.

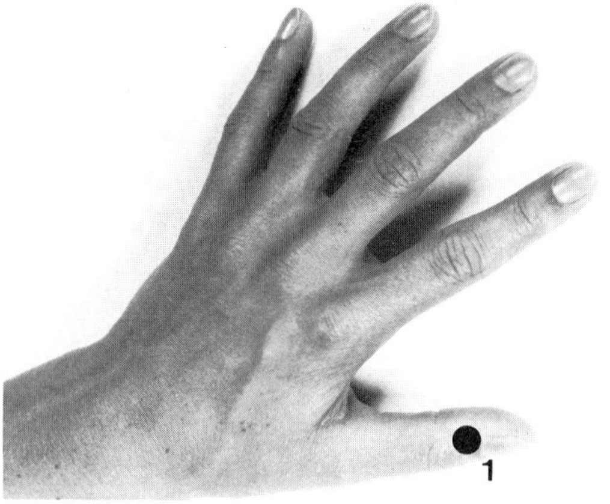


**Point 1** (Ly. 1) Left and right
Located on the lateral side of the thumb, approx. 2 mm away from the angle of the nailbed

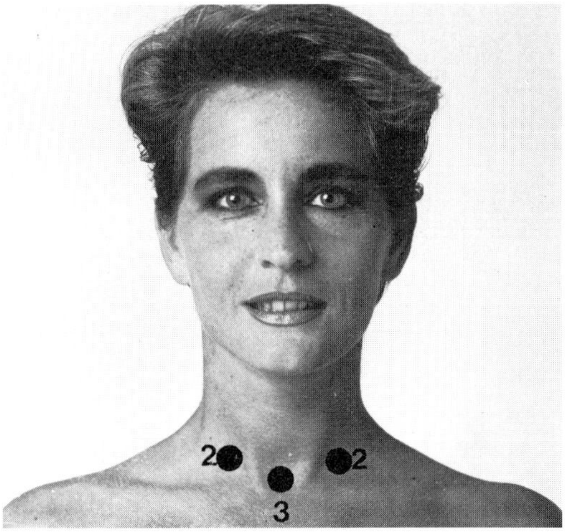


**Point 2**
(Ly. 11) Left and right
Located on the neck in the slight hollow above the collar-bone.

**Point 3**
(C.V. 22)
Located in the hollow of the neck above the breastbone.

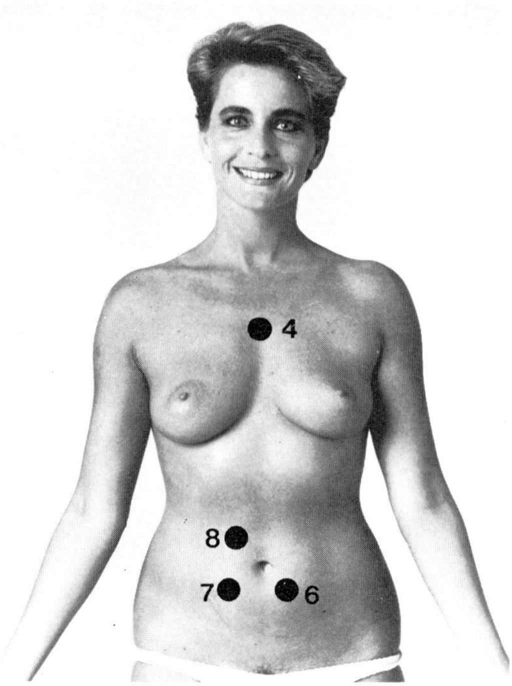


**Point 4**
(C.V. 18)
Located at the center of the breastbone at the height of the 3rd intercostal space.

**Points 6,7,8**
(Aggressive points) around the navel
By drawing a line diagonally across the navel, the first point a) can be found 2 fingerbreadths to the lower left of navel; point b) is 2 fingerbreadths to the lower right of the navel and point c) is 2 fingerbreadths to the upper right of the navel. Start with point a) on the left and follow with points b) and c) on the right.

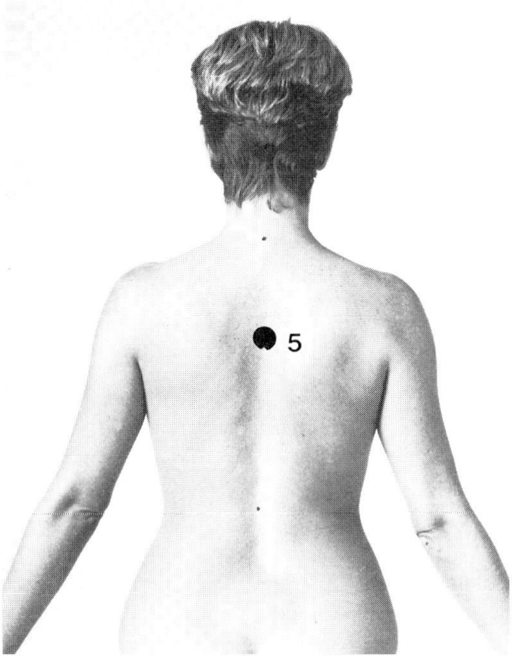


**Point 5**
(G.V. 18)
This point is located exactly opposite point 4 (C.V. 18) on the spine.

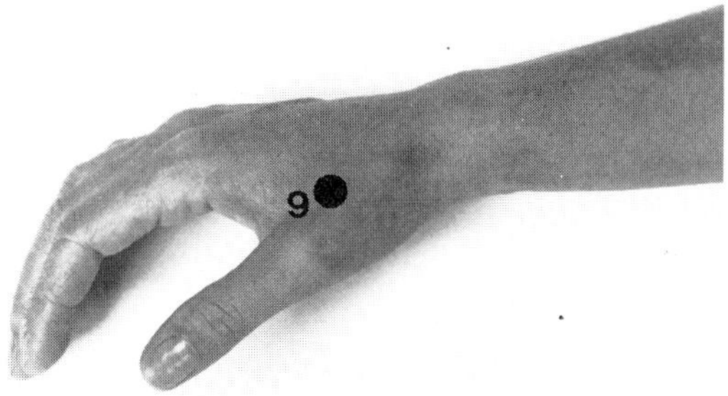


**Point 9**
(L.I. 4) Left and right
Located on the medial side of the forefinger in the angle where the metacarpal bones of the thumb and forefinger meet.

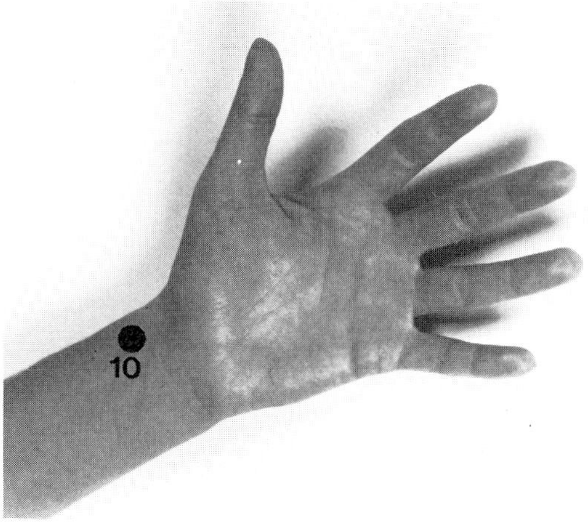


**Point 10**
(Lu. 7) Left and right
Located about 2 fingerbreadths from the 1st wrist fold in the so-called radial groove.

Here, again, use the illustrations to find the position of the points.

Even acute states of pain of unknown cause can disappear spontaneously by following this procedure. Whatever the case, this combination is an excellent form of energy treatment for preventing our bodies from being adversely affected by many sources of stress and strain.

# Regulating the Control Functions of the Brain

The human brain is still one of the greatest mysteries of life. Although much is already known about its structure, its functional centers and its forms of communication, there is still little clarity about the continual simultaneous processes that take place within this organ. We have gained a large degree of insight into the functioning of neural communication on the periphery and have also located certain centers which determine our lives. Nevertheless, we know little about the esoteric connection of mind, body and spirit. It has not been possible to find an organ or section of the brain which is responsible for energetic communication; nevertheless, reknowned scientists have postulated a large number of theories and hypotheses. Woitersdorf, for instance, is of the opinion that information is not only carried from the brain to the periphery and vice versa by neural impulses but also by electrons, and that this is carried out almost instantaneously. In the course of his research, the well-known scientist Dr. Popp has also been able to prove that our cells emanate light. They do so in a stable manner in the case of healthy cells, but in the case of sick ones, emanation increases drastically. According to Einstein's theory of photons and the findings of Hertz and Compton, photons are without mass and require some kind of vehicle in order to spread in a controlled manner. Compton proved Hertz's assumption that when light strikes matter, electrons are dispersed. The wavelength of these photons determines the rate of acceleration. Such findings were the impulse for developing Colorpuncture and form the basis of all colored-light treatment. If, therefore, photons and electrons are involved in the information system of our being, certain centers in our brains must be able to read these messages and react directly to them.

Information leads naturally to reaction – also in our bodies. Without wishing to delve too deeply into the matter in this context, we can theoretically postulate that areas of the brain beneath the pons possess the capacity to register and react to such information. At some stage in the future, the existence of such centers will certainly be proved, thus demonstrating the nature of the whole energetic system.

As we know, hormones are of vital importance. Life would be impossible without these substances which are permanently present in our blood. The centers controlling these hormones are the hypothalamus and the hypophysis. These control nutrition, circulation and metabolism, the salt and water content of the body and individual growth and maturity. It is, therefore, quite clear how important a balanced hormone system is and that in the case of irregularities, a way must be found to harmonize it. This so-called endocrine system also plays an important role when considering the controlling mechanisms of the brain. There are many more such systems, but it would exceed the scope of this book to attempt to list and explain them all. However, we can proceed on the assumption that the functions of our cells and organs are monitored and controlled by centers in the brain which require feedback from the periphery. The polarity of above and below gives rise to the image of a pyramid, with the "boss" of the controlling organs, as yet unknown, presiding at the top. Whatever the case, the transmission of information takes place in a hierarchic manner. Any kind of irregularity must therefore prompt us to reflect upon the control mechanism of the brain. All that we see, hear or feel, consciously or unconsciously, requires information and inevitably calls forth reaction. Consequently, the entire control system of our brain has to be maintained in a necessary.

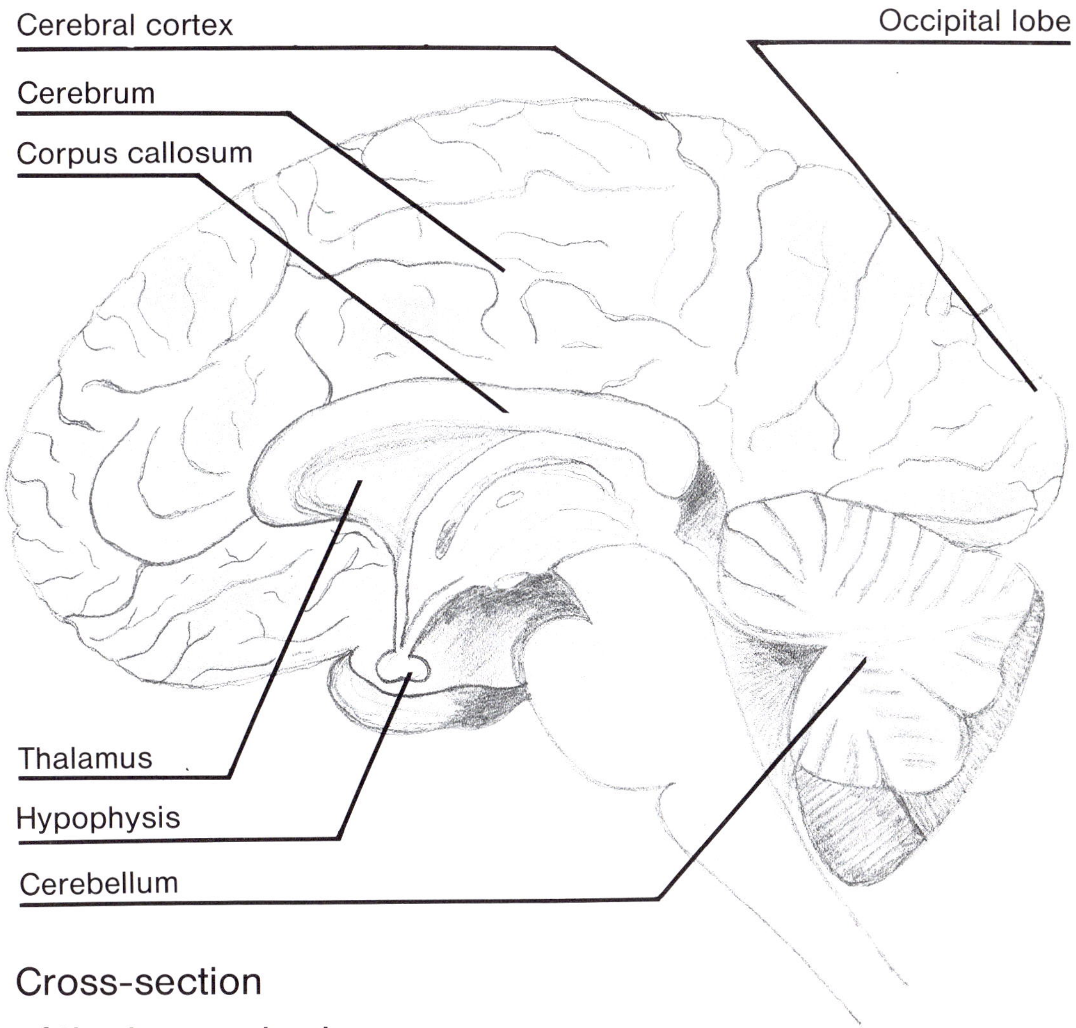


Cross-section
of the human brain

state of alertness in order to monitor the functioning of billions of cells.

In the course of my work with energetic phenomena by means of EEA, I have found a series of point combinations which influence this controlling area. By means of Kirlian photography I have been able to verify the results of this work in thousands of cases. They prove not only that manipulation of these combinations will improve the patient's subjective state, but also that negative phenomena occurring in the EEA picture can be eliminated. Long-term experiments with the acu-impulsor show that a number of these points have a harmonizing effect on the controlling mechanisms, and thus on the human organism, without involving any danger or side effects. Frequently, symptoms disappear which have nothing to do with the indications of the points being treated. This has led to the emergence of a fundamentally new form of therapy which is in no way oriented towards individual organs or symptoms; instead, emphasis is placed on the harmonization of cerebral functioning. I have termed these new procedures "control therapies", since they are directed at balancing the many and frequently complex cerebral processes. These should be carried out alternately once a week. If you has already been diagnosed by a doctor or licensed health practitioner, can apply both combinations alternating daily to support the healing process, regardless of the nature of the sickness. Ten impulses should be applied per point according to the number sequences. For the sake of simplicity, I have termed the two proposed treatments "Control I" and "Control II".

**Control I**

Treatment points 1–6, one after the other, with ten impulses each once a week as a preventive measure. This will harmonize physiological cerebral control. This is particularly recommended in the case of stress situations or nervous states. In the latter case it is recommended that the treatment be conducted daily as described.

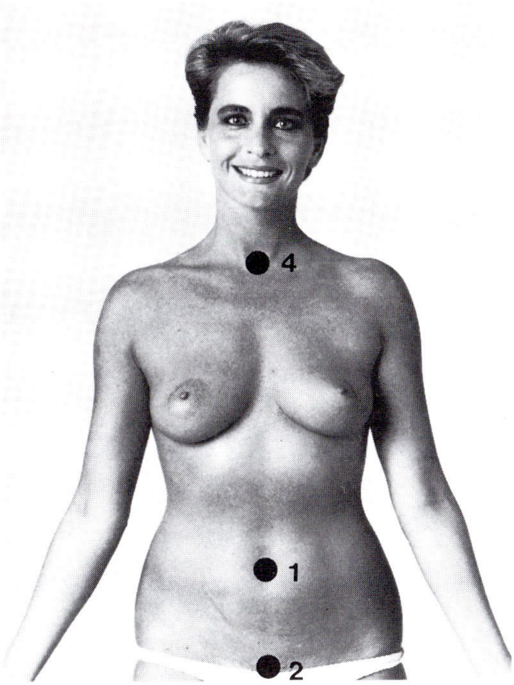


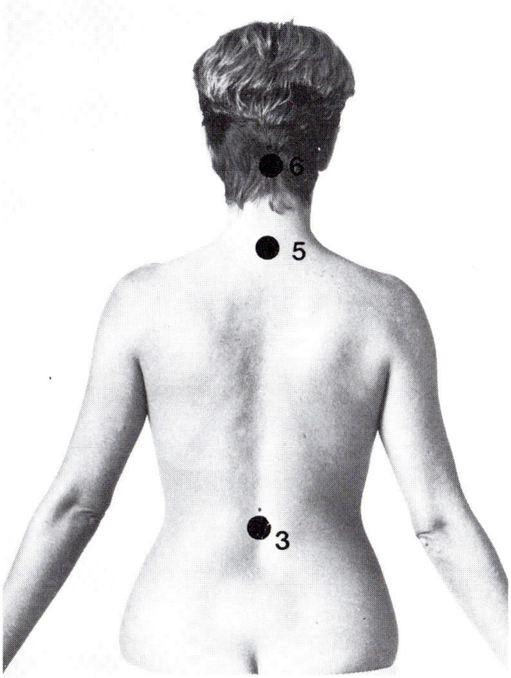


**Point 1**
(C.V. 8)
Located directly in the center of the navel.

**Point 2**
(C.V. 3)
Located 2 fingerbreadths above the pubic bone.

**Point 3**
This point is located directly opposite point 1 (C.V. 8) on the spine.

**Point 4**
(C.V. 22)
Located in the hollow of the throat above the breastbone.

**Point 5**
(G.V. 13)
Located at the end of the spinal process of the 7th cervical vertebra.

**Point 6**
(G.V. 16)
Located in the slight hollow between the 1st cervical vertebra and the skull.

## Control II

This combination also has a stimulating effect on the brain, particularly on the controlling organs. The points should be treated in the given order with the acu-impulsor, starting with the points on the left hand side. Example: Point 1 left, point 1 right, then point 2 left, point 2 right, etc.

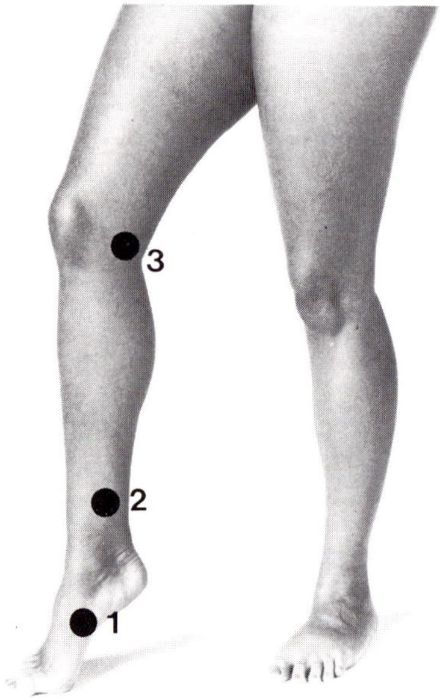


**Point 1**
(P. 4) Left and right
Located on the inside of the foot, slightly beneath the end of the first metatarsal bone.

**Point 2**
(P. 6) Left and right
Located three fingerbreadths above the medial malleolus on the medial margin of the shin bone.

**Point 3**
(Liv. 8) Left and right
Located on the posterior medial side of the knee joint gap, directly behind the tendon which can be felt at this point.

Control II can also be applied for minor ailments. It should be alternated in a daily rhythm with Control I. When the symptoms decrease, the intervals between treatments should gradually be increased until one reaches a weekly rhythm, alternating Control I and Control II.

Three alternatives for energy balancing have now been described, of which the first can be applied daily. The second involves the immune system, the lymphatic system, and strength in general. The third alternative has the function of regulating overall controlling mechanisms. Applied early, i.e. in times without pain and sickness, all three can be regarded as a true form of prophylaxis.
In the course of the book, it is my intention to propose ways of helping yourself in the case of everyday ailments and in order to eliminate painful states quickly. I have been guided by my experience with patients in my practice, whom I always give "homework" to do, for without a person's will to recover, even the very best forms of therapy are futile. It is therefore essential for sick people to play an active part in overcoming their illness so that they can regain their position as full members of society and their immediate circle. A healthy person can apply the acu-impulsor as a means of preventing disease. However, never forget that any kind of ailment should first be diagnosed by a doctor or licensed health practitioner.

# TREATMENT OF THE LYMPHATIC SYSTEM

1. Lymph Rhombus
2. Points Located on the Head which Act on the Lymph System
3. Improving the Lymphatic Flow via the Lymph Glands of the Neck
4. Improving the Flow of Lymph from Above to Below
5. The Abdominal Rhombus

Apart from the ways of balancing energy in the lymphatic system already described, there is also a series of important point combinations. These relate to specific ailments. Lymph treatment is a vital part of natural therapeutics. The following combinations serve to support other forms of treatment, such as medication, acupuncture and the use of injections. Spinal and joint disorders, rheumatic troubles, rhinitis, sinusitis and certain types of headache all respond very well to the treatment of the lymphatic points listed here. As has already been mentioned, I always include lymph treatment when dealing with illnesses and ailments in my practice. Besides using the acu-impulsor, I also recommend additional fast-acting therapy which addresses itself to the entire organism.

The following points are indicated for shoulder/arm tension, pain in the back of the neck, a tingling sensation in the fingers and as an additional means of treatment for dyspnea. Each point is given 10 impulses. Repeat after 5 minutes.

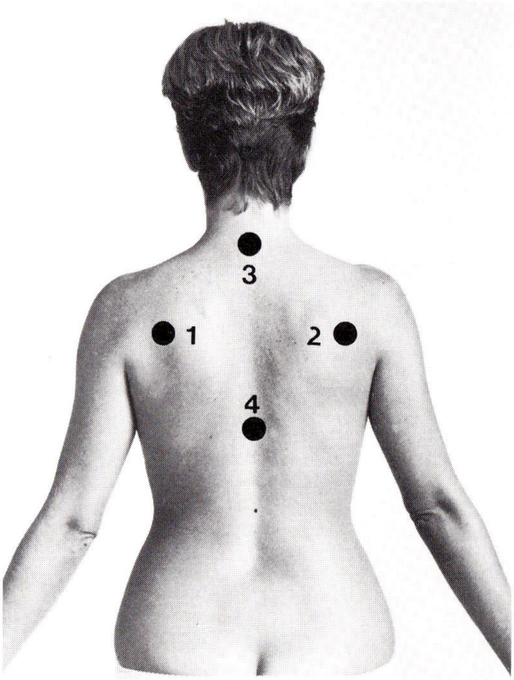


**Points 1 + 2**
(S.I. 11) Left and right
Located in the middle of the shoulder blade, below a palpable ridge of bone.

**Point 3**
(G.V. 13)
Located directly at the end of the spinal process of the seventh cervical vertebra.

**Point 4**
(G.V. 6)
Located directly on the spinal process of the 11th dorsal vertebra.

There are five points which can be used for treating lymphatic congestion of the head. They are effective in cases of rhinitis, sinusitis and inflamed mucous membranes of the nose, lymph congestion and the resultant headaches.

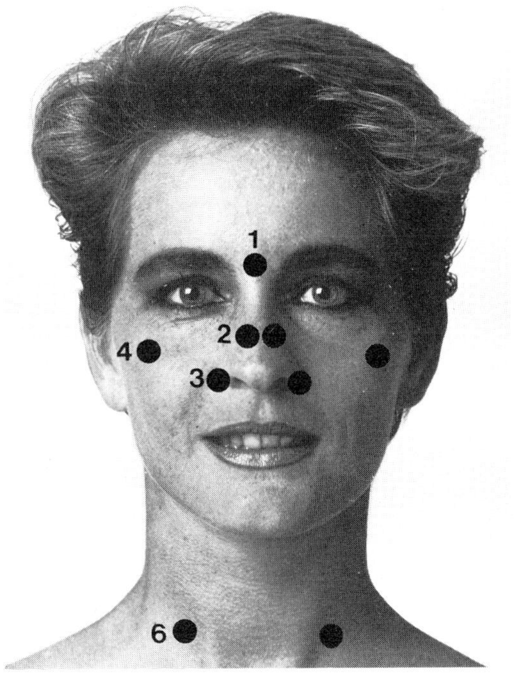


**Point 1**
(Yin trang)
This point is located exactly between the eyebrows.

**Point 2**
Cartilage point
Located in the middle of the nose where the cartilage begins.

**Point 3**
(L.I. 20) Left and right
Located at the side of the nose, a few millimeters from the naso-labial fold.

**Point 4**
(S.I. 18) Left and right
Located on the cheekbone, where a small hollow can be felt below the outer corner of the eye.

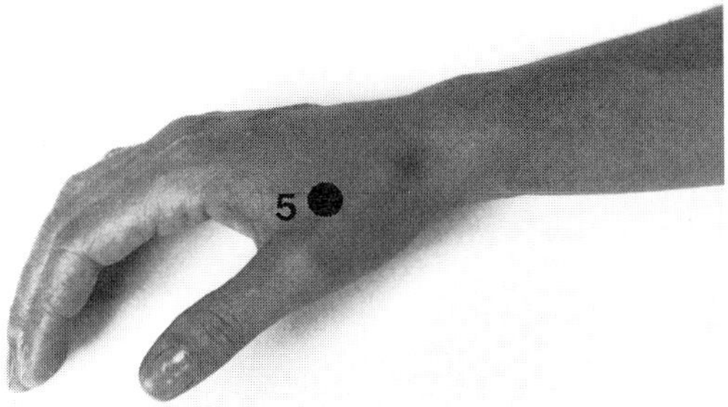


**Point 5**
(L.I. 4) Left and right
Located on the medial side of the forefinger in the angle where the metacarpal bones of thumb and forefinger meet.

**Point 6**
(Ly. 11) Left and right
Located on the neck in the slight hollow above the collar-bone.

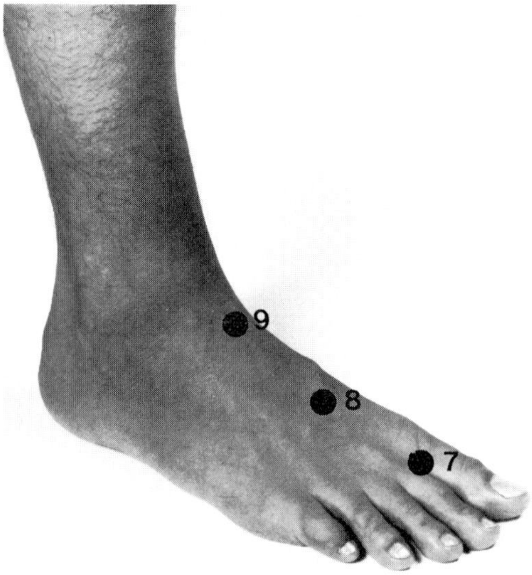


In accordance with the basic principles of acupuncture, points on the opposite pole of the body must also be treated. These are three pairs of points on the top of the foot.

**Point 7**

(Ly. Foot A) Left and right
Located in the fold between the 1st and 2nd toes.

**Point 8**

(Ly. Foot B) Left and right
Located on the middle of the foot on a line running upwards from point A.

**Point 9**

(Ly. Foot C) Left and right
Located in the bend of the foot joint

All the points listed should be treated with 10 impulses each in the given order. The program should be repeated after 5 minutes.

**COMBINATION I**

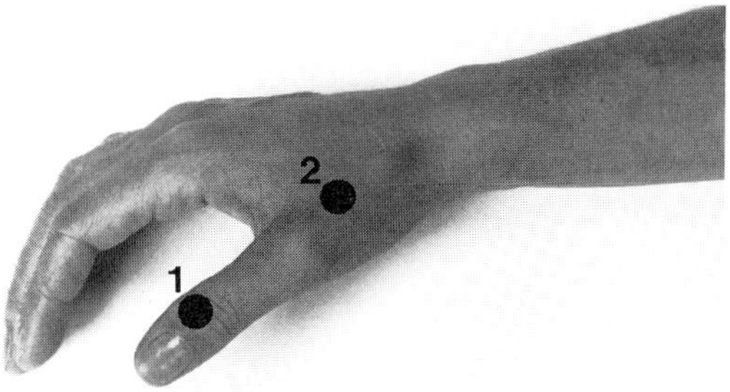


**Point 1**
(Ly. 1) Left and right
Located laterally on the thumb, 2 mm away from the angle of the nailbed groove in a diagonal direction.
**Point 2**
(L.I. 4) Left and right
Located on the lateral side of the forefinger in the angle where the metacarpal bones of thumb and forefinger meet.

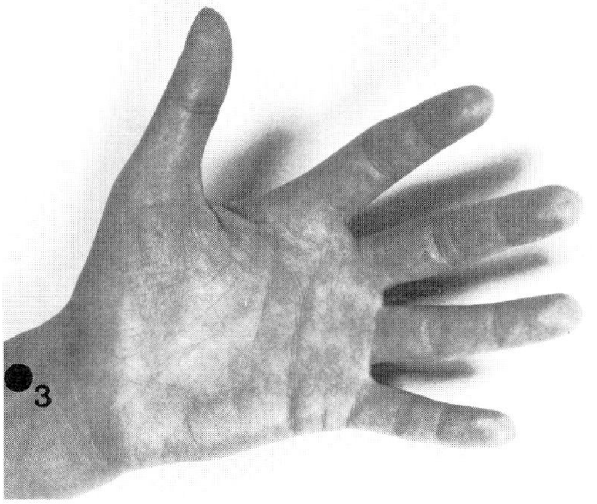


**Point 3**
(Lu. 7) Left and right
Located about 2 fingerbreadths from the first crease of the wrist in the so-called radial groove.

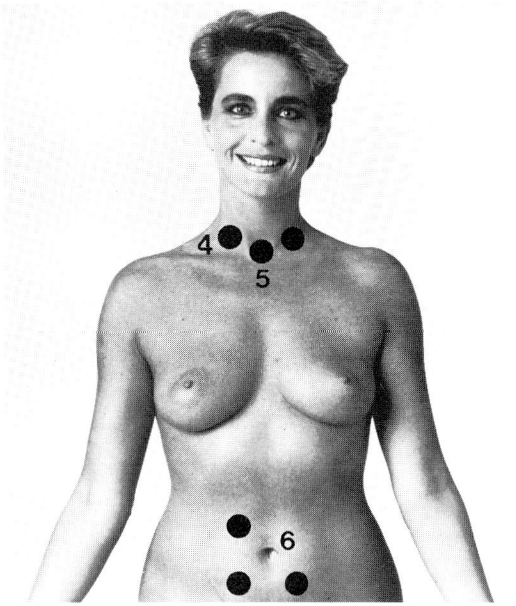


**Point 4**
(Ly. 11) Left and right
Located in the small hollow above the collar-bone.
**Point 5**
(C.V. 22)
Located in the hollow above the breastbone.
**Point 6** (Aggressive zones)
Draw two diagonal lines over the navel. The first point is situated on the diagonal line, 2 fingerbreadths to the left below the navel. The second point is located to the right, in the same manner; the third point is situated on a diagonal line 2 fingerbreadths to the right above the navel.
The combination is particularly suitable for children who suffer from constant swelling of the lymph glands on the neck. Ear troubles and descending bronchial catarrh can be also be improved. Apply 10 impulses per point and repeat once.

**COMBINATION II**

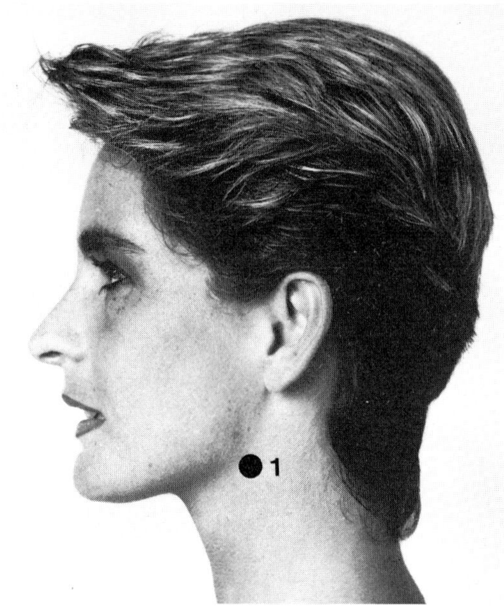


**Point 1**
(Tonsillar point) Left and right
Located between the angle of the jaw bone and the neck.

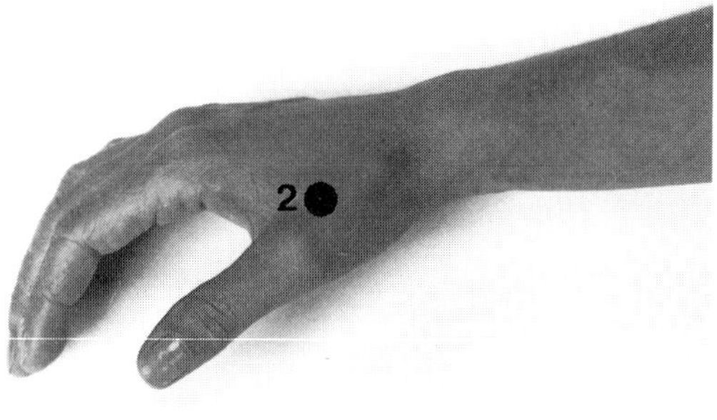


**Point 2**
(L.I. 4) Left and right
Located on the lateral side of the forefinger in the angle where the metacarpal bones of the thumb and forefinger meet.

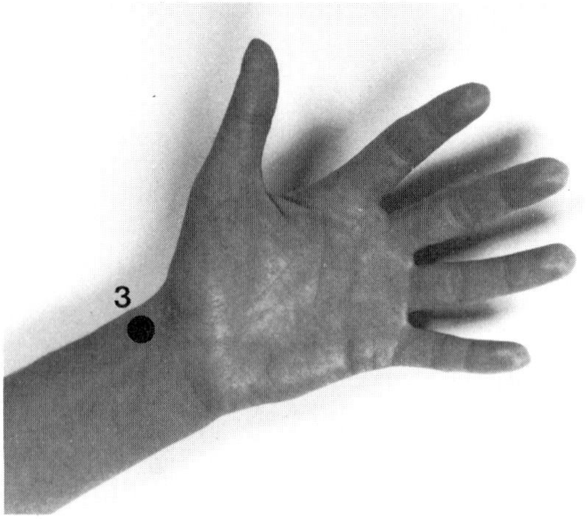


**Point 3**
(Lu. 7) Left and right
Located about 2 fingerbreadths from the 1st wrist crease in the so-called radial groove.

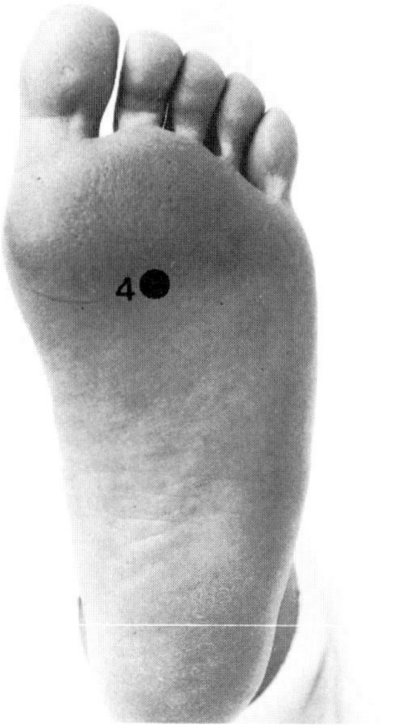


**Point 4**
(K. 1) Left and right
Located on the sole of the foot, between the ball of the big toe and the ball of the little toe.

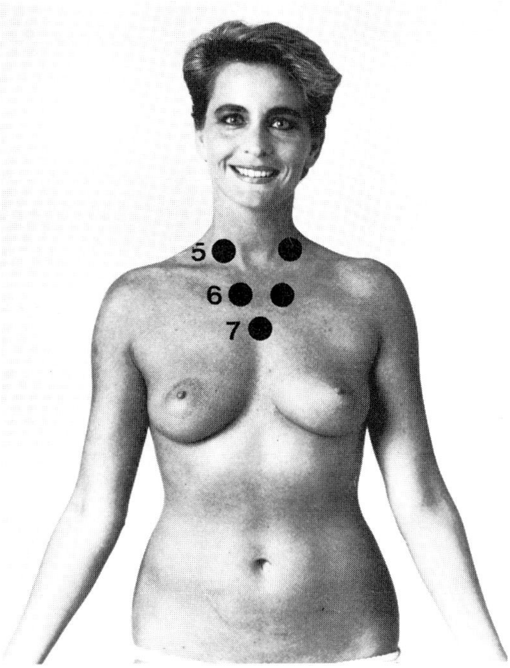


**Point 5**
(Ly. 11) Left and right
Located in the small hollow above the collar-bone.

**Point 6**
(K. 27) Left and right
Located at the point on the lower edge of the collar-bone where it forms a joint with the breastbone.

**Point 7**
(C.V. 18)
Located in the middle of the breastbone at the height of the 3rd intercostal space.

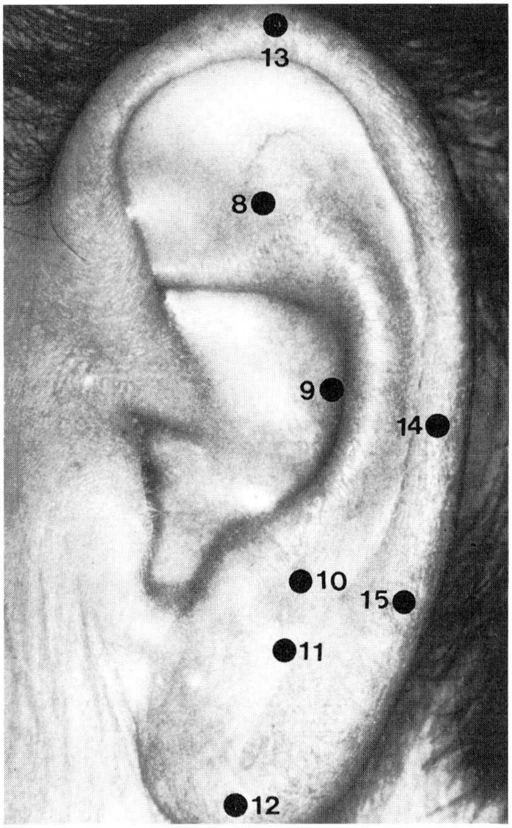


**Ear points:** 8 – 9 – 10 – 11 – 12 – 13 – 14 – 15

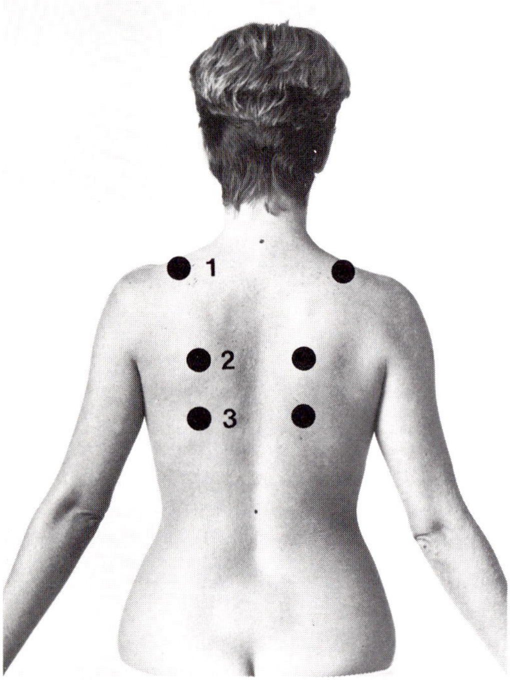


**Point 1**
(T.H. 15) Left and right
Located on the shoulder in the middle of the top edge of the trapezius muscles.

**Point 2**
(U.B. 41) Left and right
Located between the 6th and 7th ribs, a handsbreadth from the midline of the body.

**Point 3**
(U.B. 42) Left and right
Located between the 7th and 8th ribs, a handsbreadth from the midline of the body.

One very good way of promoting the flow of lymph came to light in the course of treating pain. It involves the specific arrangements of four points in four areas of the body. The points are arranged in a rhombus form and are to be found on the chest and in the abdominal, pelvic and dorsal regions. As already stated, they are particularly to be recommended for pain of all types. In my opinion, the lymphatic system plays an important role in all types of pain, meaning that the rhombuses can be treated for the prevention of pain and as a supporting measure in the treatment of acute illness. Ten impulses per point should be applied in the given order, and then repeated once.

This combination should be applied for congestion in the lower abdomen and minor pelvis.

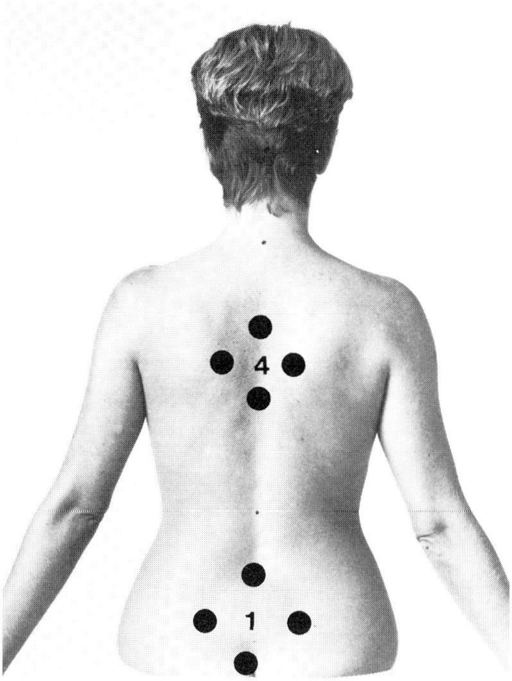


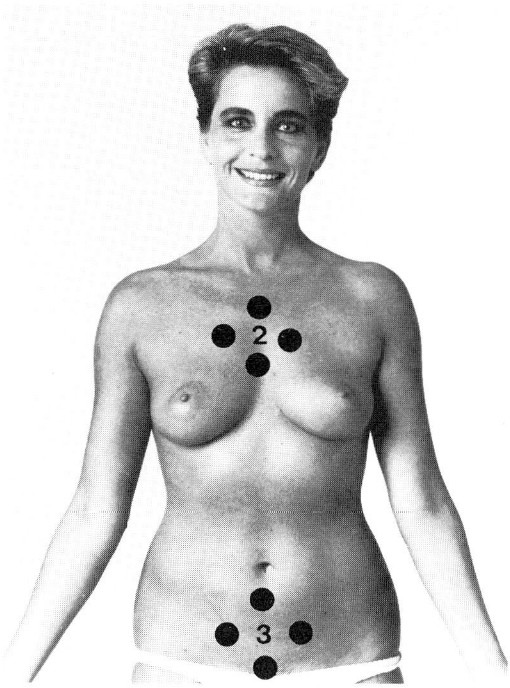


**Point 1** (Pelvic Rhombus)
The points are located at the beginning of the anal crease at the transition from the sacrum to the transition of the 5th lumbar vertebra, to the left and right on the iliac crest.

**Point 2** (Breast Rhombus)
This point lies on the line drawn between the left and right axillar fold. Start with the point in the middle of the breastbone. All the points are 2 fingerbreadths apart.

**Point 3** (Abdominal Rhombus)
The top point is positioned 2 fingerbreadths below the navel and the botom one is on the edge of the pubic hair. The points to be treated are the ones on the right and left. These are positioned at the same distance as the top and bottom points.

**Point 4** (Life Rhombus)
The central point is located on the spine on line with the middle of the shoulder blade. The four points surround it 2 fingerbreadths away.

Lymphatic congestion is a frequent disorder today. Pain or pressure in the pelvic organs, complaints of the spine, or headaches rising from the back of the neck are all indications for rhombus treatment.
The following treatment plan has proved successful in practice and can be applied alternately:

a) a combination of the pelvic and chest rhombus;
b) a combination of the abdomen and thorax rhombus.

Both combinations have a decongesting effect. The lymphatic flow is released and the energy balance can re-establish itself.

# Headache and Migraine

1. Basic Combination
2. Headaches Rising from the Back of the Neck
3. Headaches Occurring at the Crown of the Head
4. Pains in the Temples
5. Psychological Tension
6. Sensation of Dullness in the Head

Millions of people all over the world suffer unpleasant headache both occasionally or daily.
These range from dizziness, pressure, and a burning sensation in the eyes to the most awful forms of migraine, accompanied by nausea, sensitivity to light and extreme pain. The abuse of pain-killers is a serious matter because all pain-killers have side effects in the long run and they do not treat the root causes of the pain. The best they can do is interrupt the vicious circle of suffering.
With regard to these unpleasant disorders, I therefore consider it of the utmost importance to give a detailed account of the ancient knowledge of acupuncture, segmental therapy and reflexotherapy. By regulating the energy potential with the help of the acu-impulsor, it is certainly possible to reduce medication. By localizing the headaches and complaints, we can begin to deduce the causes. For instance, headaches and migraines which rise up from the back of the neck correspond to the uro-genital tract. Pains at the vertex have their root causes in the abdomen. Pains in the right area of the forehead indicate liver or gall bladder disorders, while the left area of the forehead is connected with the pancreas and the intestines. Pains in the middle of the forehead can be caused by acute or chronic sinusitis, or alternatively, they may be an indication of stomach disorders. Always remember that headaches can have much more serious causes, such as arteriosclerosis or other forms of strain on the blood vessels, or even tumors. Therefore, do not treat yourself for headaches for a long time without consulting a doctor or licensed health practitioner first.

I have discovered various combinations of points which form a basic framework for treating headaches.

The following combinations always constitute the beginning of headache therapy. They are usually very effective in the case of troublesome pains. Nevertheless, depending on the localization or the type of headache, I have developed individual programs to be applied additionally. In acute cases, one should begin with the basic combination. This usually causes the pains to disappear or at least become considerably alleviated. In the last case one can then, depending on the localization, go on to apply the individual specific programs. Following the numerical order given, ten impulses should be given to each point. Where necessary, the treatment may be repeated once or twice. In time, the intervals between the headaches should increase, making the specific procedures superfluous. During pain-free times, carry out the energy balancing programs, alternating programs I and II. It is sufficient to do this once or twice a week. You can now begin to free yourself of these troublesome pains which are such a handicap in life.

Begin impulse treatment at the points farthest away from the head. Then treat the hand points and the ear points and finish off with the points on the head. Apply ten impulses to each point in a one second rhythm.

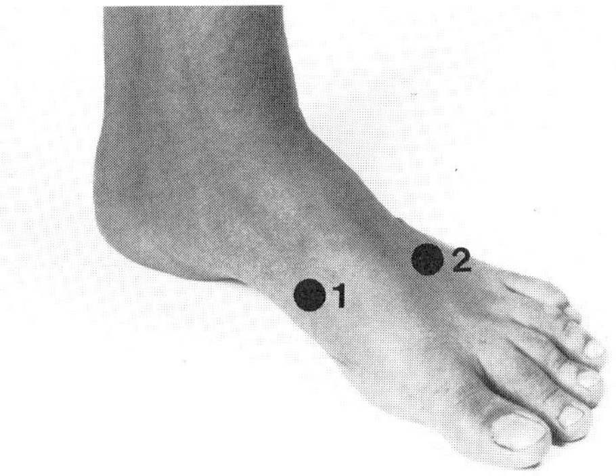


**Point 1**
(P. 4) Left and right
Located on the inside of the foot, slightly below the end of the 1st metatarsal bone.

**Point 2**
(Foot reflex zone point for the gallbladder) On the right hand side only
This point is located on the top of the foot on the line between the 4th and 5th toes at the end of the metatarsal bone.

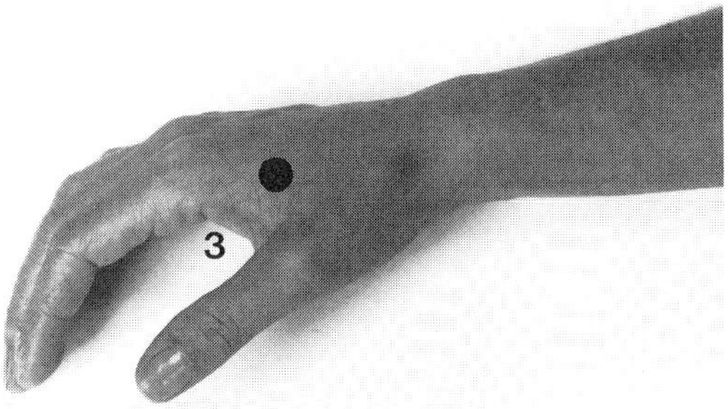


**Point 3**
(Hand point: forefinger) Left and right
Located 2 fingerbreadths behind the base joint of the index finger. This point will be found to be very painful

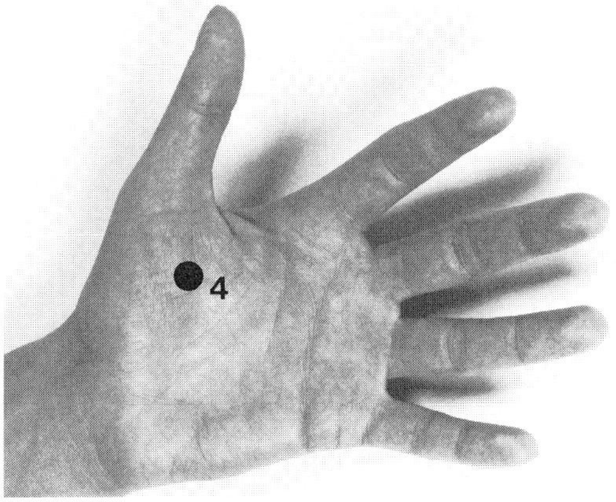


**Point 4**
(Hand point: ball of thumb) Left and right
This point is located in the middle of the ball of the thumb and will be found to be very painful.

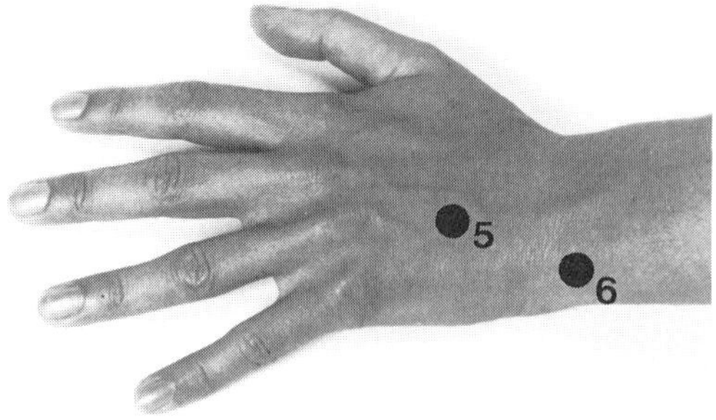


**Point 5**
(Psyche point) At the back of the left hand
This point is situated between the 4th and 5th fingers, at the point where the metacarpal bones end.
**Point 6**
(Circulation point)
This point is on the outer side of the wrist.

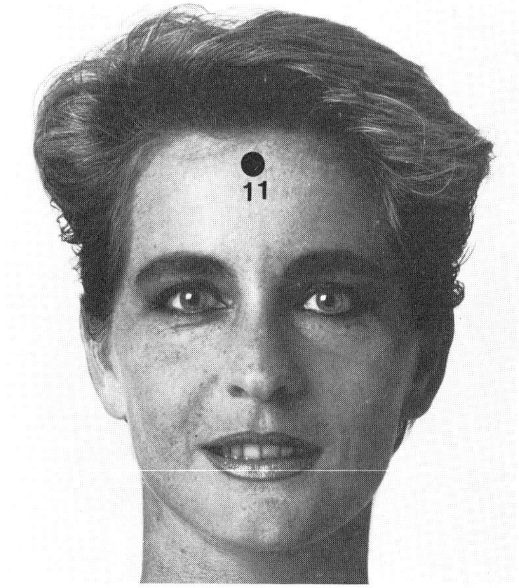


**Point 11**
Located in the middle of the forehead, 1 fingerbreadth below the hairline

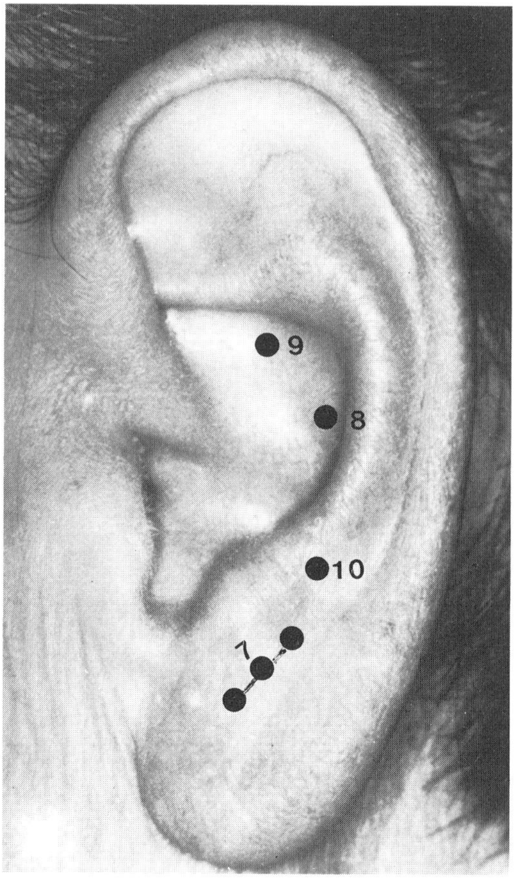


**Point 7**
(Ear point) The headache line in the ear
**Point 8**
(Ear point) Liver point
**Point 9**
(Ear point) Kidney point
**Point 10**
(Ear point) Neck point

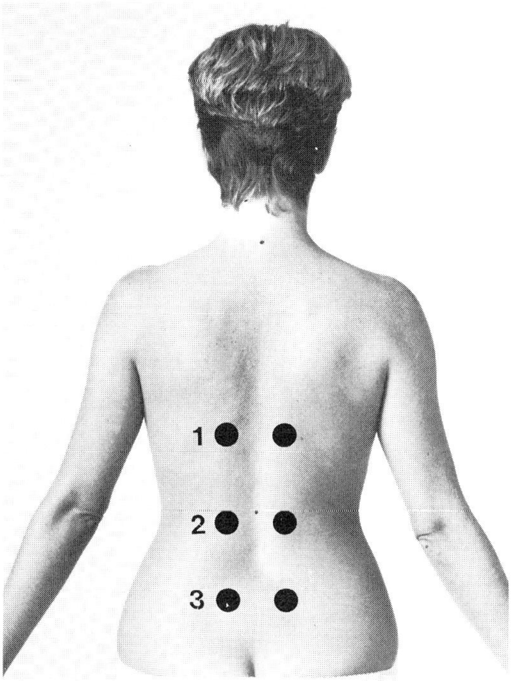


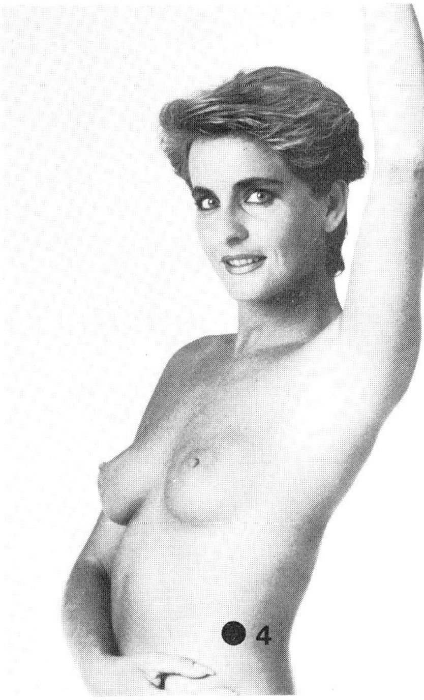


**Point 1**
(U.B. 18) Left and right
Located between the 9th and 10th ribs, 2 fingerbreadths from the center of the body.

**Point 2**
(U.B. 23) Left and right
Located between the 2nd and 3rd lumbar vertebrae, 2 fingerbreadths from the center of the body.

**Point 3**
(U.B. 31) Left and right
Located on the inner side of the sacral canal.

**Point 4**
(G.B. 25) Left and right
Located at the free end of the 12th rib.

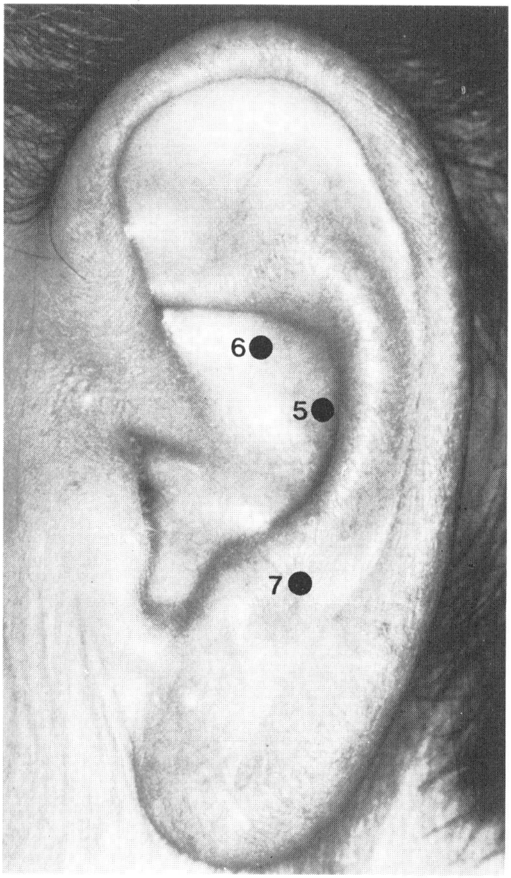


**Point 5**
(Ear point) Liver
**Point 6**
(Ear point) Kidney
**Point 7**
(Ear point) Neck

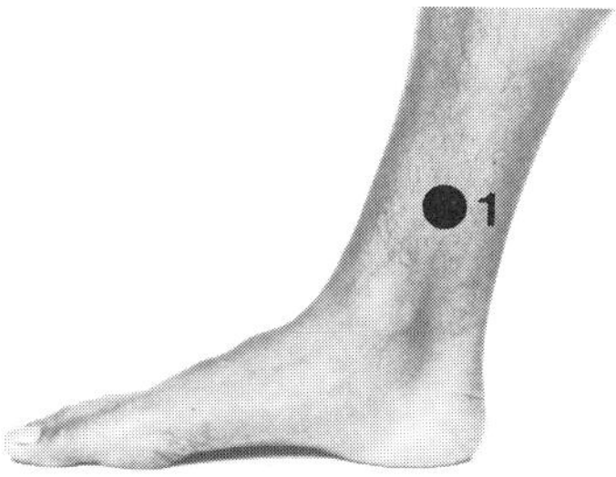


**Point 1** (P. 6) Left and right
The points are located approximately 3 fingerbreadths above the medial malleolus on the inner edge of the shin bone.

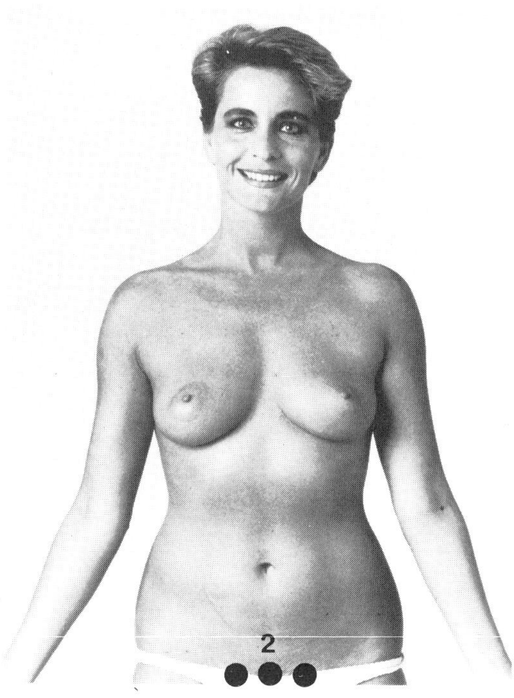


**Point 2** (Kundalini Line)
All three points are located directly on the pubic hair-line. The middle point is beneath the navel and the other two are approx. 2 fingerbreadths to the left and right of it.

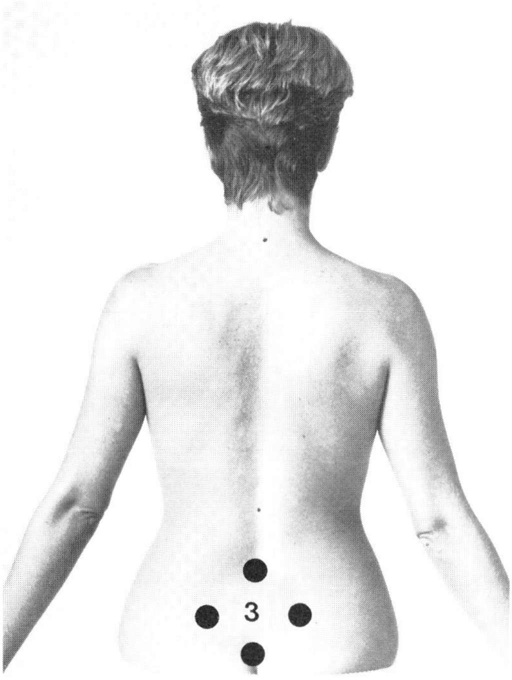


**Point 3**
(Pelvic rhombus)
The points are located at the beginning of the anal crease, at the transition between the sacrum and the 5th lumbar vertebra, and to the left and right on the iliac crest.

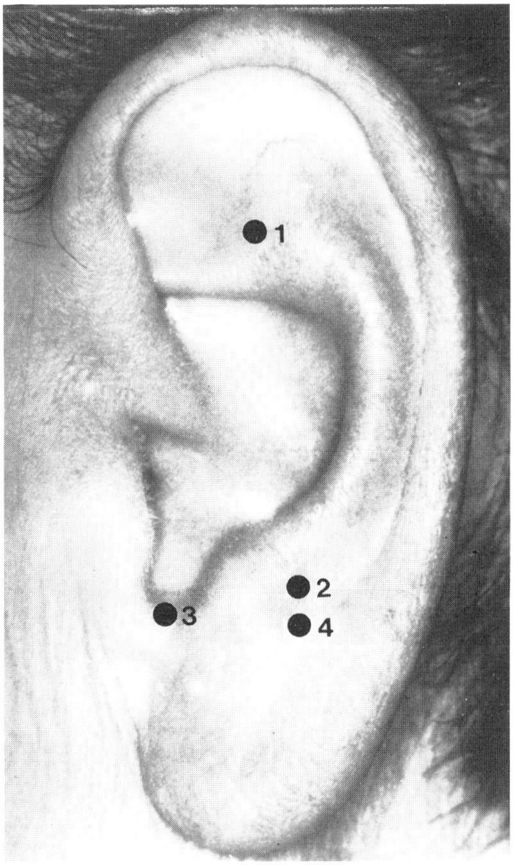


**Point 4**
Ear points 1 - 4

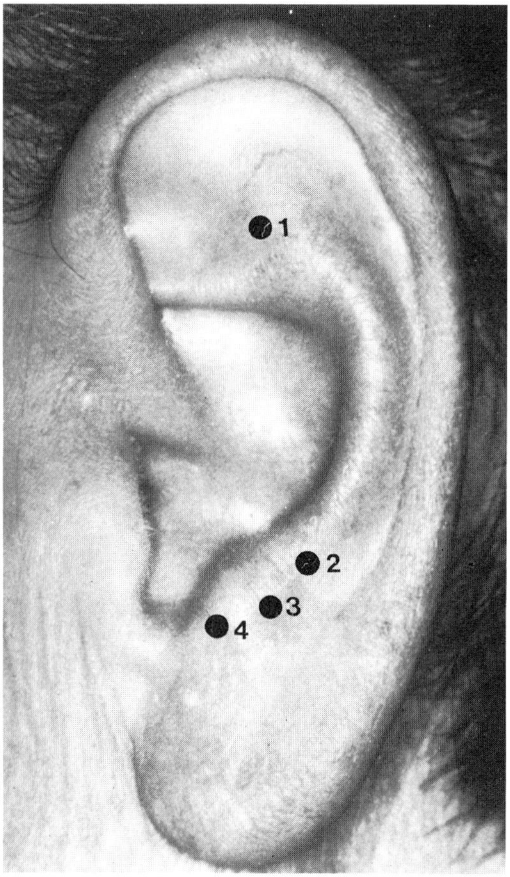


**Point 1:** Ear point
**Point 2:** Ear point
**Point 3:** Ear point
**Point 4:** Ear point

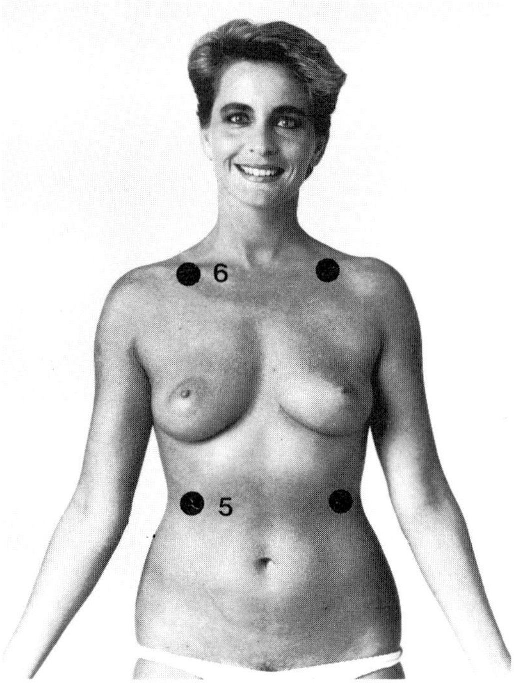


**Point 5**
(Li. 13) Left and right
Located on the 11th rib at a slight distance from the lateral end.

**Point 6**
(St. 12) Left and right
Located on the upper margin of the collarbone in line with the nipples and about 4 fingerbreadths from the midle line of the body.

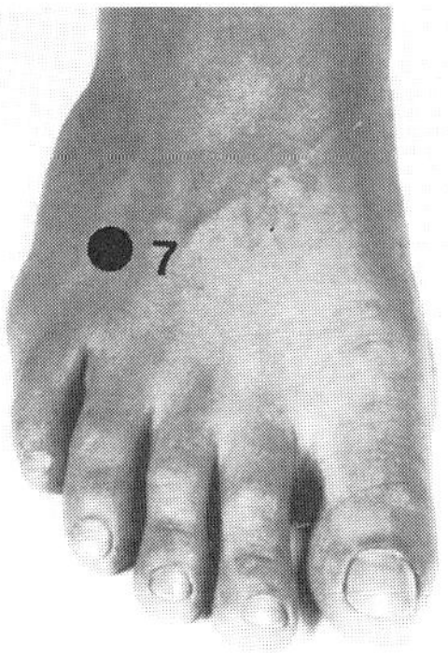


**Point 7**
(Foot reflex zone G.B.) On the back of the right foot
This point is located on the line between the 4th and 5th toes, at the point where the metatarsal bones end.

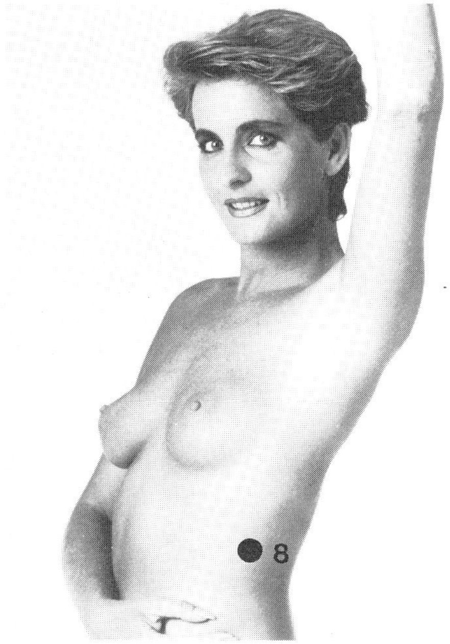


**Point 8**
(G.B. 25) Left and right
Located on the free end of the 12th rib.

Headaches due to stress or mental and emotional unease are extremely widespread. Especially those people who know that their nervous system is weak and who are inclined to react to all kinds of worry with tension in the head should regularly treat the following combinations of points in the given order. The control therapies I and II listed under "Energy Balancing" have proved to be very successful in this respect. These therapies have a generally relaxing effect and, in the long term, they will stabilize the psyche.

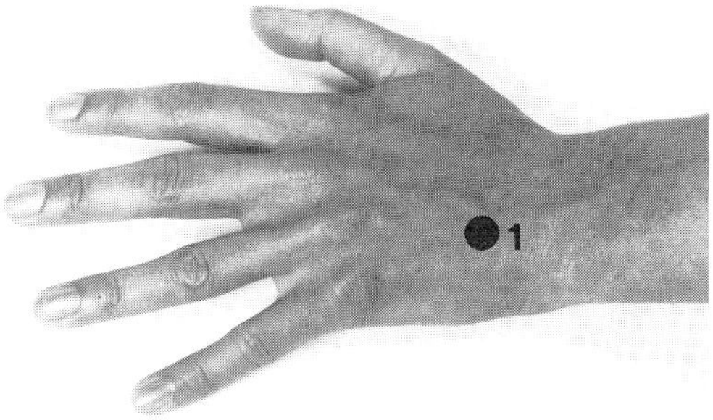


**Point 1**
(Psyche point on the Left hand)
Located at the point between the 4th and 5th fingers where the metacarpal bones end.

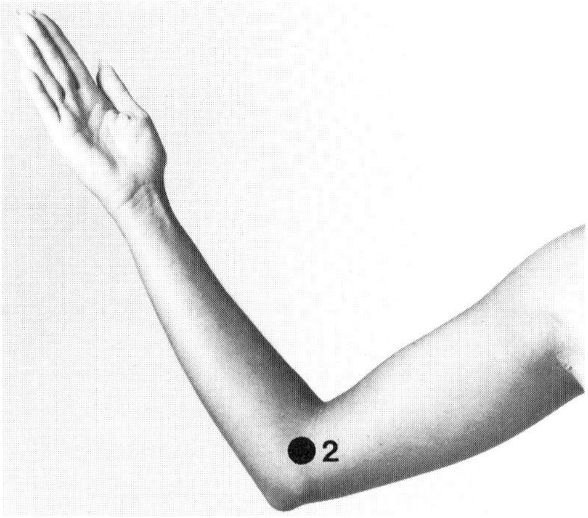


**Point 2**
(H. 3) Left and right
Located at the exterior end of the elbow crease.

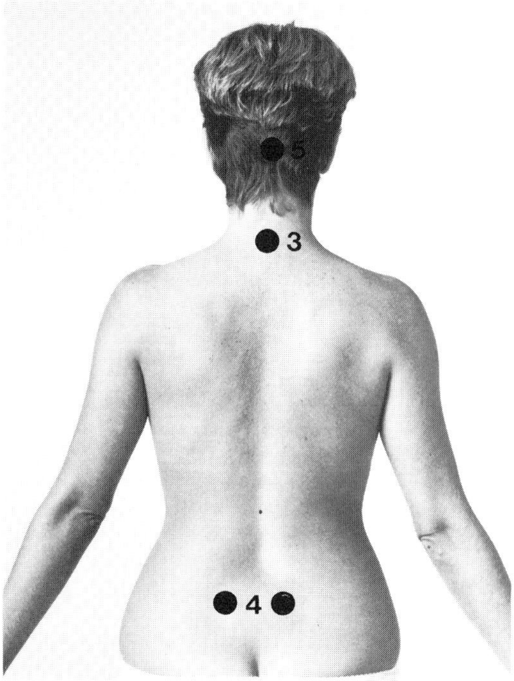


**Point 3**
(G.V. 13)
Located at the tip of the spinal process of the 7th cervical vertebra.

**Point 4**
(U.B. 31) Left and right
Located on the medial side of the 1st sacral canal.

**Point 5**
(G.V. 16)
Located in the slight hollow between the 1st cervical vertebra and the skull.

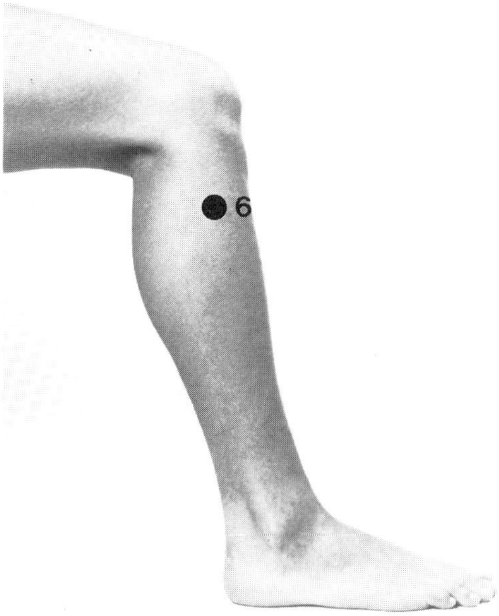


**Point 6** (St. 36) Left and right
Located on the front of the leg, 3 finger-breadths below the knee in the middle of the shin. This point can also be found by placing the palm of the hand on the knee-cap. The tip of the middle finger will then lie directly on the point in question.

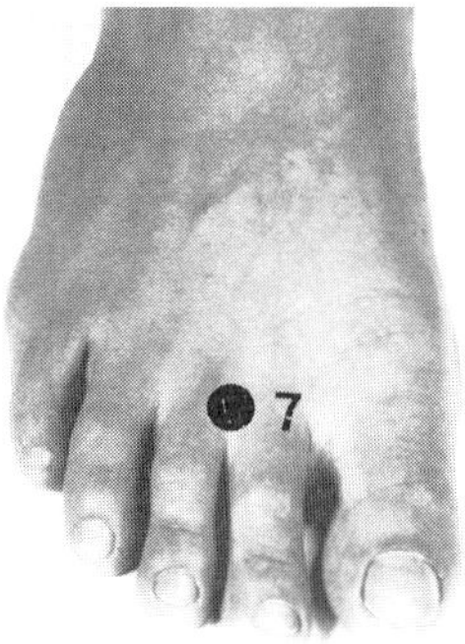


**Point 7** (St. 44) Left and right
Located on the lateral side of the 2nd toe beside the basal joint.

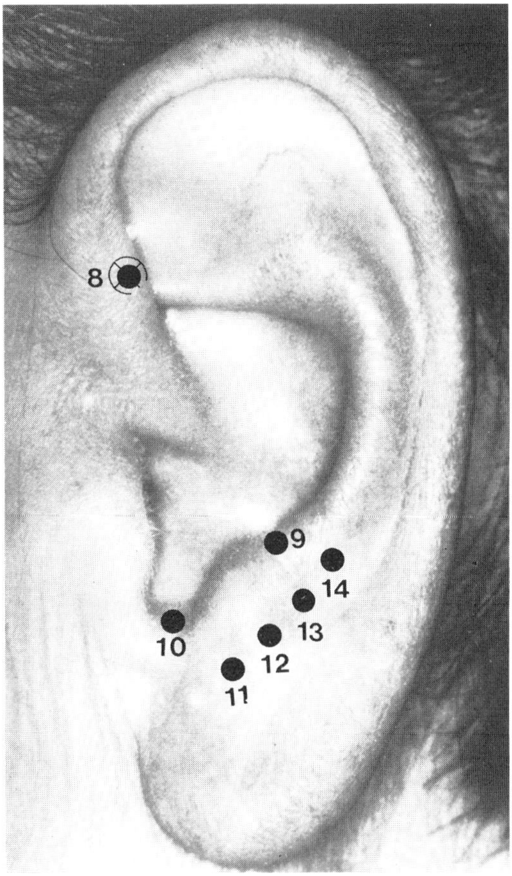


**Point 8** (Ear point)
**Point 9** (Ear point)
**Point 10** (Ear point)
**Point 11** (Ear point)
**Point 12** (Ear point)
**Point 13** (Ear point)
**Point 14** (Ear point)

As a rule, a sensation of dullness in the head is caused by disturbances in the flow of lymph from the head. Congestion in the blood supply may also be found. In the latter case, 10 impulses per point should be applied daily and repeated once or twice.

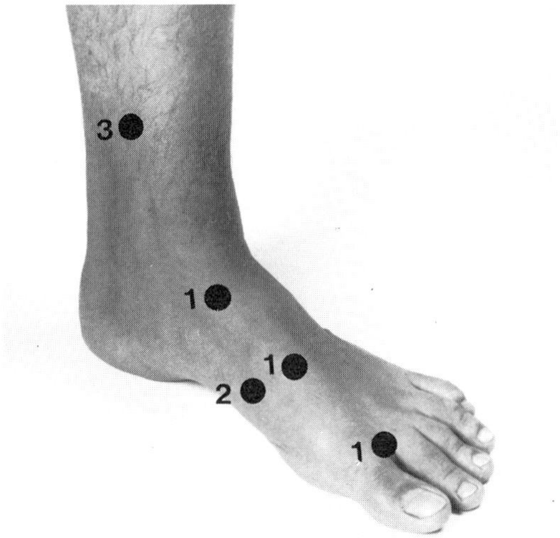


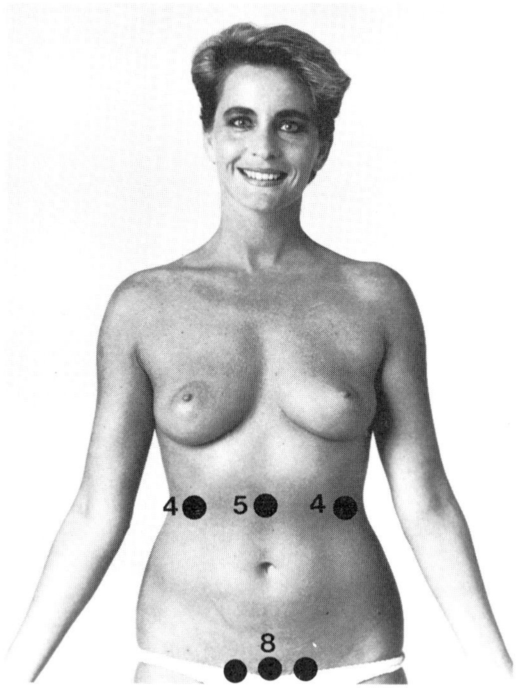


**Point 1**

(Lymph zones A–C) Left and right

A) is located in the fold between the 1st and 2nd toes.

B) is located on the line in the middle of the foot leading upwards from from point A.

C) is located in the bend of the ankle joint.

**Point 2**

(P. 4) Left and right

Located on the medial side of the foot, slightly below the end of the metatarsal bone.

**Point 3**

(P. 6)

Located approx. 3 fingerbreadths above the medial malleolus on the inner margin of the shinbone.

**Point 4**

(Liv. 13) Left and right

Located on the 11th rib, at a slight distance from the lateral end.

**Point 5**

(C.V. 12)

Located at the center of an imaginary line connecting the end of the breastbone and the navel.

**Point 8**

(Kundalini Line)

A) is located on the pubic hair line, below the navel.

B) is 2 fingerbreadths to the right of point A.

C) is 2 fingerbreadths to the left of point A.

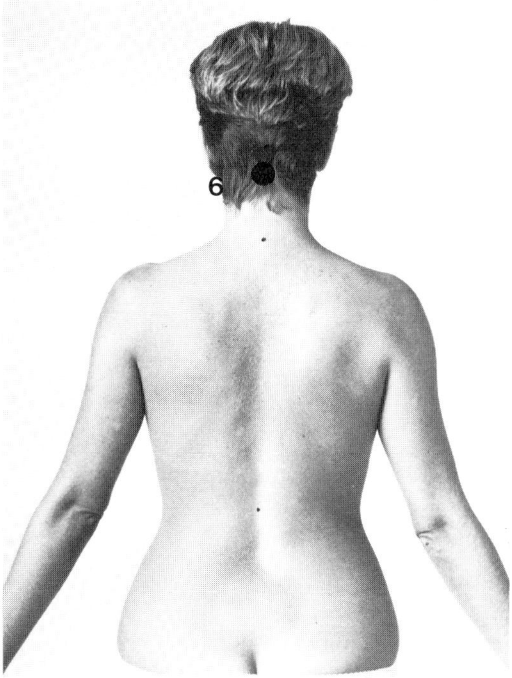


**Point 6**
(G.V. 15)
Located directly on the tip of the spinal process of the 2nd cervical vertebra.

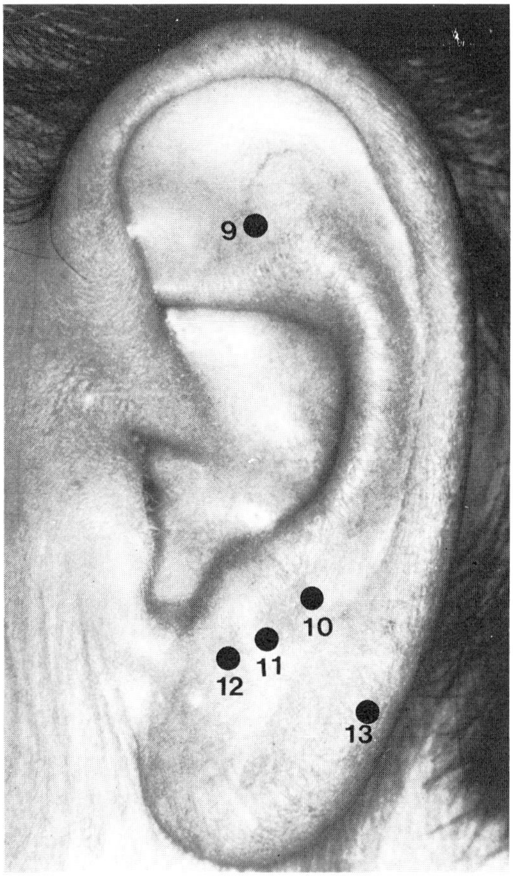


**Point 9** (Ear point)
**Point 10** (Ear point)
**Point 11** (Ear point)
**Point 12** (Ear point)
**Point 13** (Ear point)

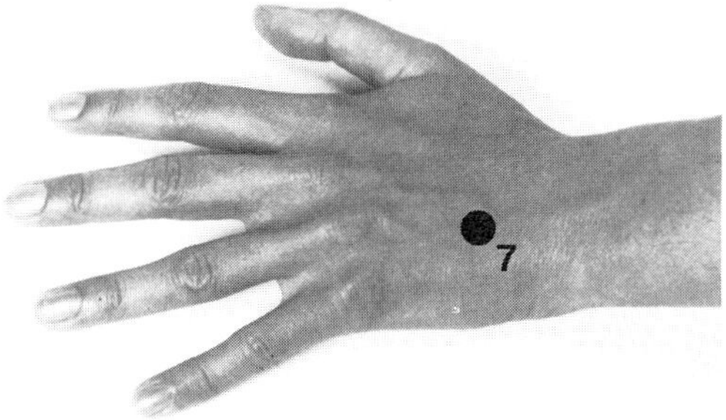


**Point 7**
(Psyche point) Back of left hand
Located between the 4th and 5th fingers where the metacarpal bones end.

There are a number of additional measures that can be carried out to support this treatment. Among them are such simple things as warm compresses on the liver or kidneys or – for women before and after their period – warmth applied to the lower lumbar region of the spine and to the sacral area.

No-one has to suffer headaches. It often takes only three to four months of energy balancing for headaches to be cleared away for good. In the case of migraine, however, it frequently takes longer. Nevertheless, by taking painkillers, all you do is gain momentary relief. The headaches will return, maybe for life. Seen in this light, the simple use of the acu-impulsor and the little time involved put it at an advantage over all kinds of manipulative treatment.

# Complaints of the Spine

1. Pain in the Cervical Spine
2. Pain in the Thoracic Spine and in the Shoulder Region
3. Pain in the Lumbar Spine

Complaints of the spine are almost as common as migraine. Individual symptoms may range from lumbago to the most severe forms of sciatic and neuralgic pain which may even extend to the arms. When dealing with these complaints, the close relationship between the spine and the inner organs is often neglected. The spinal marrow is connected to the inner organs by the spinal nerves. Therefore, functional disturbances on an energy level may cause muscular tension in the related segments. A thorough examination of the muscular condition before initiating treatment will allow the experienced physiotherapist to detect the organs which are subject to stress and thus function in a disturbed manner. These interrelationships had already been described around the turn of the last century. Mackenzie, Head, Putkammer, Kiebeler, Mozer, Dicke and Leube, who researched and reported their findings independently of each other, were among the first scientists to explore the connections between the surface of the body and the inner organs. The results of their research play an important part in the diagnostic procedures of today. In segmental diagnosis and other methods which concentrate on the surface of the body, palpatory findings provide information on the malfunctioning of inner organs. Such dysfunctions put a strain on the spine and are, in the final analysis, responsible for causing organic damage and degenerative conditions. This is understandable in view of the fact that vertebrae and bones do not degenerate on their own and that muscular tension plays an important part in initiating and promoting such processes. From a holistic point of view, the relationship between the spine and all other parts of the body must always be given due consideration. Shortened legs, blockages of the sacral and iliac articulations, toxicosis due to foci (stemming from dental focal infection or the lymph system as a whole), false posture caused by vocational activities, and, above all, mental and psychological disturbances must also be taken into consideration. To quote W. Penzl,"The spine is the central axis of our body and personality. Any disturbance of this axis will have repercussions on our personality." This is an apt description of the role that the spinal axis plays in the interdependence of physical and psychological factors. Spinal complaints will have an adverse effect on the psyche, and vice versa. Treatment of the spine with the acu-impulsor is particularly significant since it will influence the entire body and all its functions. The combination of acu-impulsor therapy with specific exercises for the spine has proved to be of particular success and shows lasting results. I have been recommending special spinal exercises to many of my patients since as long ago as 1969. In a recent effort to enhance the effect of these exercises, a cassette has been produced with a group of excellent musicians. One side of this cassette, which is part of the Audio-Energetics Program, contains a totally new form of acoustic structures while the other provides the listener with meditative music which will help relax the spine and balance out the disturbed flow of energy. We have discovered that the three elements of acu-impulsor use, gymnastics and relaxation not only do away with pain in the spine but also provide a positive form of stimulation which will benefit all people on a physical and mental level alike. When carrying out treatment for spinal complaints, treat the following points with the acu-impulsor for ten seconds each in the given order. Then, if you have the above cassette, listen to the first side and do the gymnastics as instructed. After this, relax and listen to the second side, which will soothe and calm you on all levels of being.

In conclusion, it must be said that backache is something which can be avoided. However, it must almost be added that you should consult a doctor or licensed health practitioner before starting self-treatment in order to make sure that a serious complaint is not overlooked.

We now begin with the points for treating or soothing spinal forms of pain. Start out with the lymph treatment, the second element in the energy balancing program, and depending on where the pain is caused, continue with one of the three given combinations.

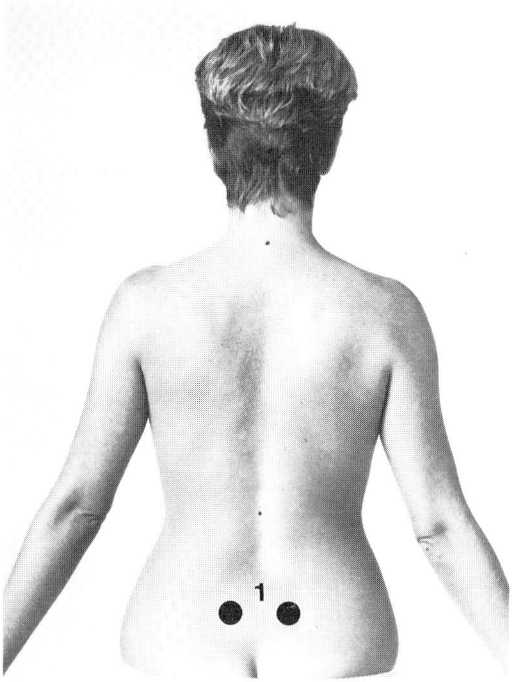


**Point 1** (Bl. 31) Left and right
Located on the medial side of the 1st sacral canal.

**Point 2**
(Lymph point of the foot) Left and right
A) is located in the crease between the 1st and 2nd toe.
B) is located on a line starting out at point A) and leading up to the middle of the forefoot.
C) is located in the crease formed at the front of the foot when you raise your toes off the ground.

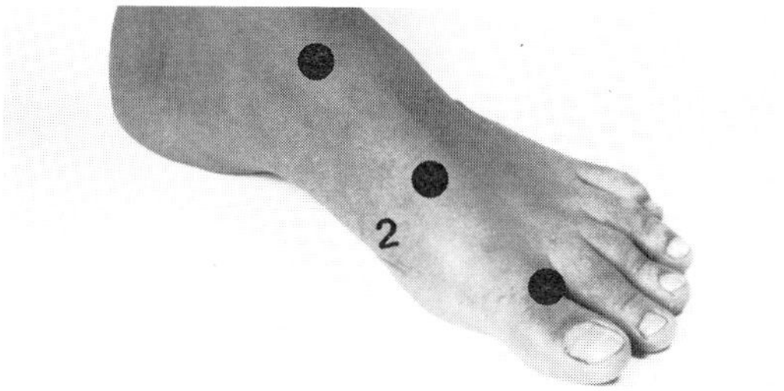

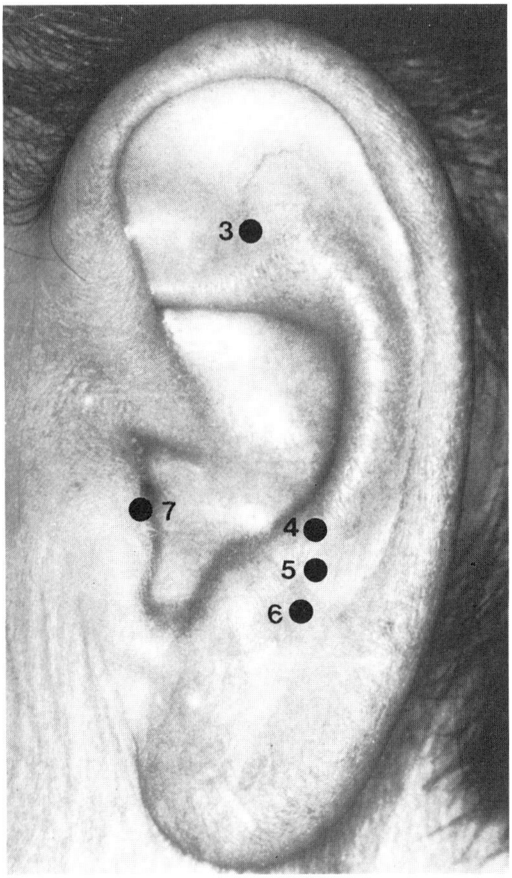


**Point 3** Ear point
**Point 4** Ear point
**Point 5** Ear point
**Point 6** Ear point
**Point 7** Ear point

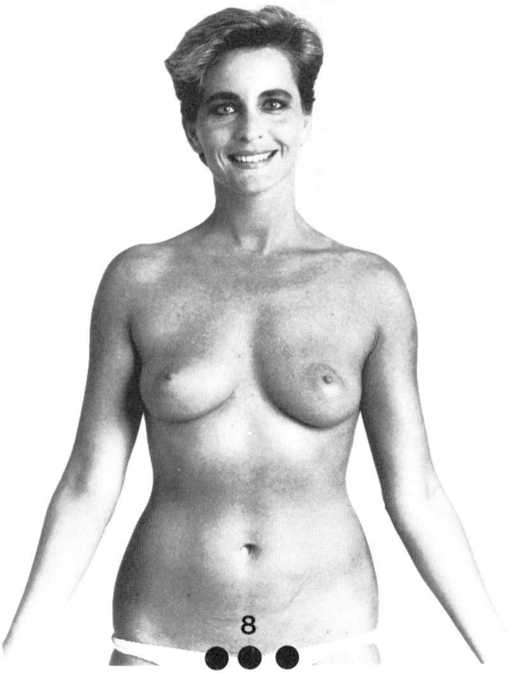


**Point 8**
(Kundalini Line)
The three points lie on the upper edge of the pubic hair.
A) is located below the navel.
B) is 2 fingerbreadths to the left of A).
C) is 2 fingerbreadths to the right of A).

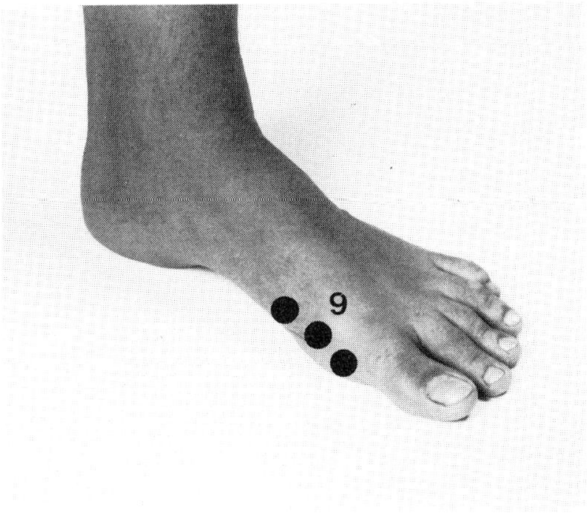


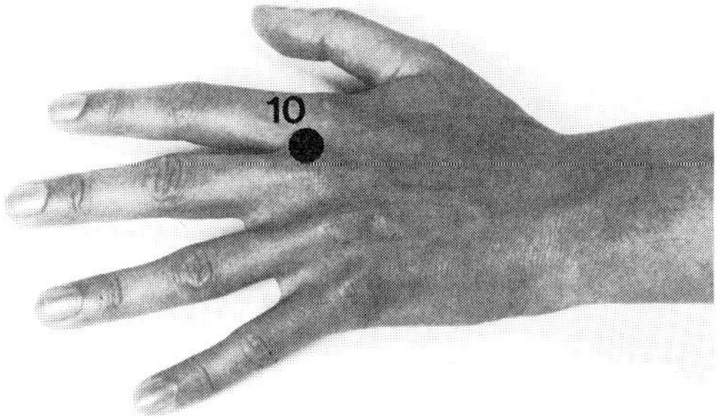


**Point 9**
(Foot reflex zone of the cervical spine) Left and right
Located near the big toe on the medial side of the foot.

**Point 10**
Positioned in the crease at the basal joint of the index finger on the lateral side of the hand. Treat both hands.

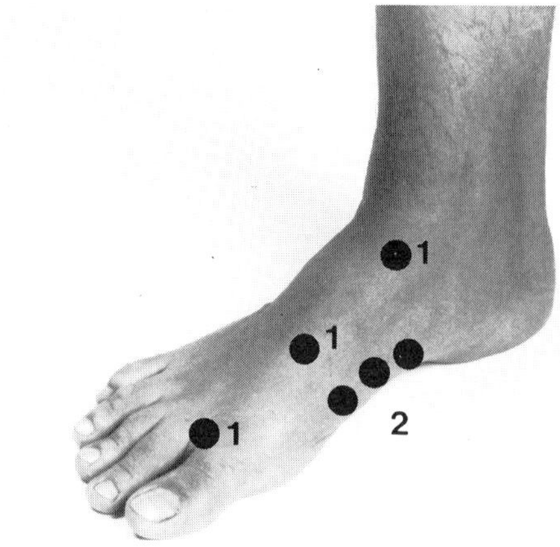


**Point 1**
(Lymph points of the foot) Left and right

A) is located in the crease between the 1st and 2nd toe.
B) is located on a line leading up from point A) to the middle of the forefoot.
C) is located in the crease formed at the front of the foot when you raise your toes off the ground.

**Point 2** (Foot reflex zone of the thoracic spine) Left and right
Located in the area where the foot arches away from the ground.

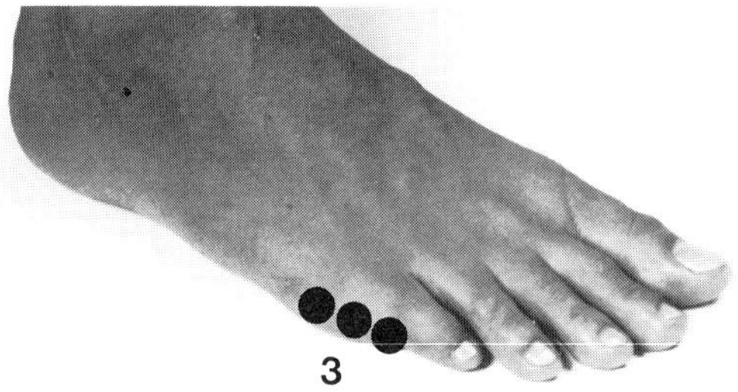


**Point 3** (Foot reflex zone of the shoulder) Left and right
Located on the lateral side of the foot, near the basal joint of the little toe.

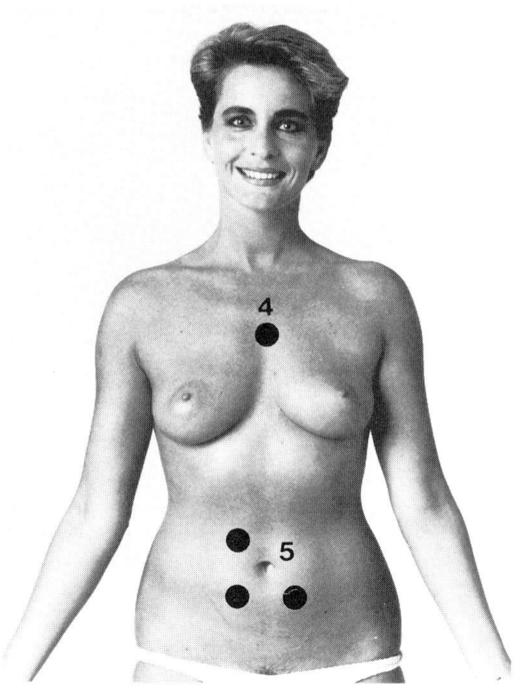


**Point 4**
(C.V. 18)
Located on the midline of the body at the height of the 3rd intercostal space.

**Point 5**
(Aggressive zones)
Draw two imaginary diagonal lines over the navel. The first point is on the line running from left to right and is located 2 fingerbreadths away from the bottom of the navel. The second point, which is also 2 fingerbreadths away from the bottom of the navel, is at the bottom of the other diagonal line. The third point is at the top of the first diagonal line, 2 fingerbreadths away from the top of the navel.

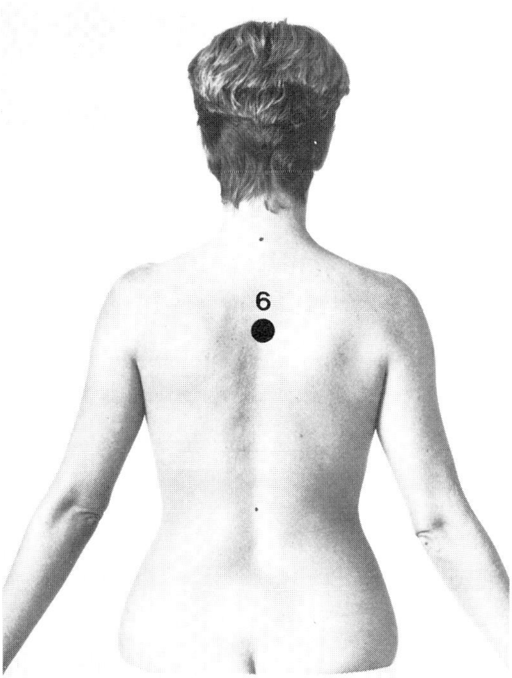


**Point 6**
(G.V. point)
Located on the spine, opposite point 4 (C.V. 18) on the chest.

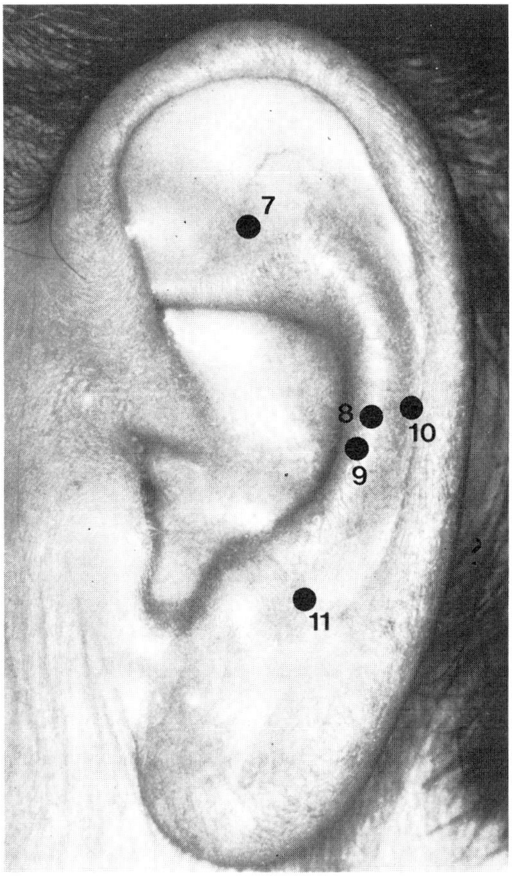


**Point 7** Ear point
**Point 8** Ear point
**Point 9** Ear point
**Point 10** Ear point
**Point 11** Ear point

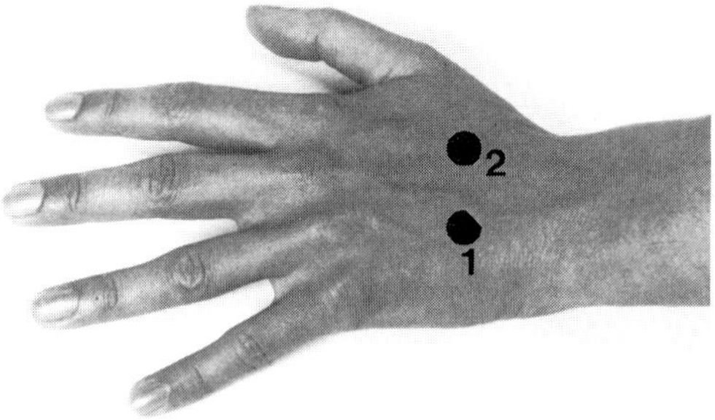


**Points 1 + 2**

(Hand points of the lumbar spine) Left and right

Both points are located on the back of the hand, point 1 lying on the line leading from between the index and the 2nd finger; point 2 lies on the line leading from between the ring and the little finger.

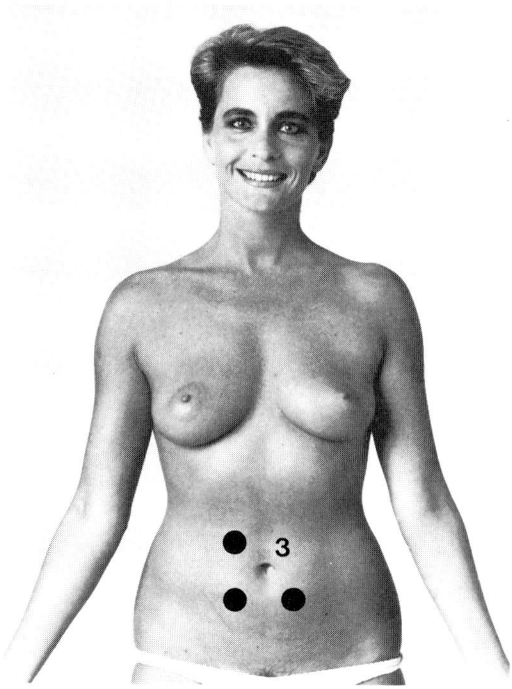


**Point 3**

(Aggressive zones)

Draw two imaginary diagonal lines over the navel.

The first point is on the line running from left to right and is located 2 fingerbreadths away from the bottom of the navel. The second point, which is also 2 fingerbreadths away from the bottom of the navel, is at the bottom of the other diagonal line. The third point is at the top of the first diagonal line, 2 fingerbreadths away from the top of the navel.

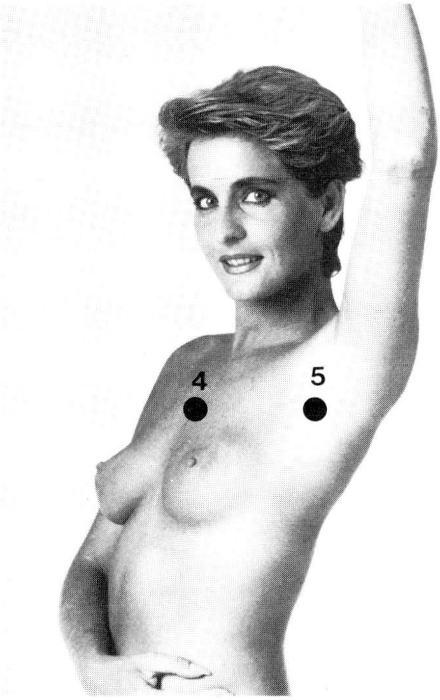


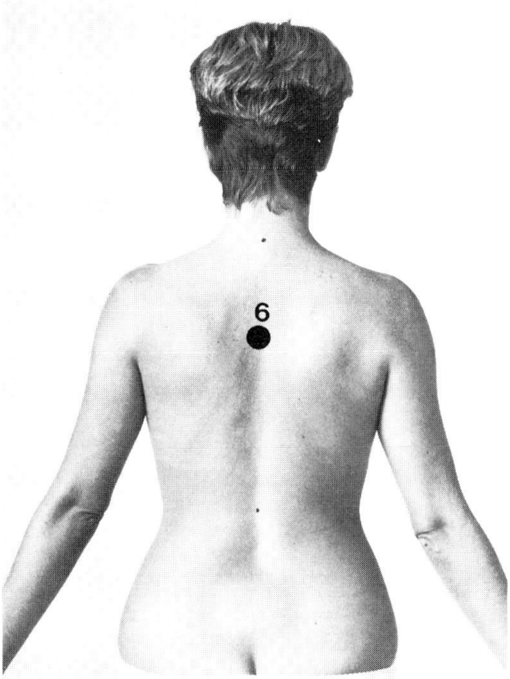


**Points 4, 5, 6 and 7**

(Point 7 is not illustrated)

Point 4 is positioned on the breastbone, at the height at the 3rd intercostal space. Draw an imaginary line from point 4 around the whole of the body, where you will find the other points. Point 5 is located in the left armpit and point 7 in the right armpit, while point 6 is positioned on the back, opposite point 4.

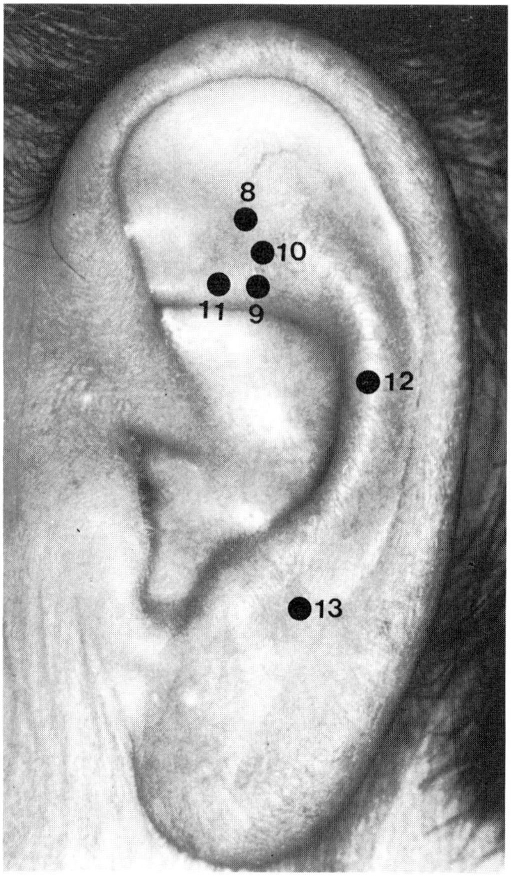


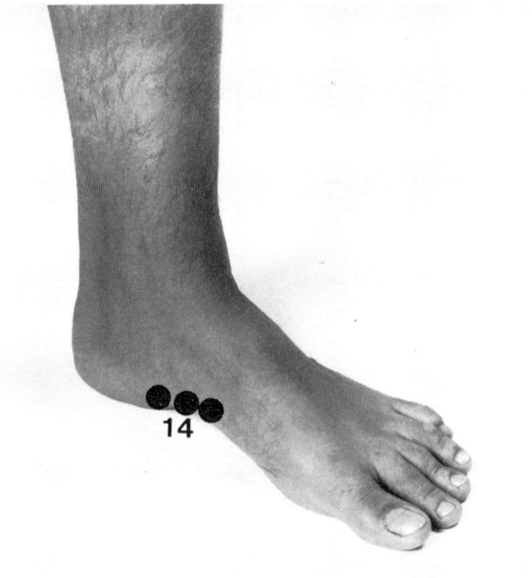


**Point 14**
Foot reflex zones of the lumbar spine
This collection of three points lies near the heel on the medial side of the foot.

**Point 8** (Ear point)
**Point 9** (Ear Point)
**Point 10** (Ear point)
**Point 11** (Ear point)
**Point 12** (Ear point)
**Point 13** (Ear point)

# Sciatica

## Neural Pain in the Legs

# Brachialgia

## Neural Pain in the Arms

Sciatica is an extremely painful complaint which can be caused by chilling, a slipped disc or even a bad tooth. Since it can also be caused by serious illnesses such as osteoporosis or cancerous metastasis, it should always be examined by a doctor or a licensed health practitioner.
Treatment with the acu-impulsor will work wonders in many cases. It will soothe the pain involved immediately, and, in some cases, will make it disappear altogether. Whatever the cause, sciatica can be treated with the acu-impulsor at the same time that diagnostic and other therapeutic measures are being carried out, making use of the following well-proved combinations. Start with the points on the pain-free side of the body and treat each one with ten impulses each.

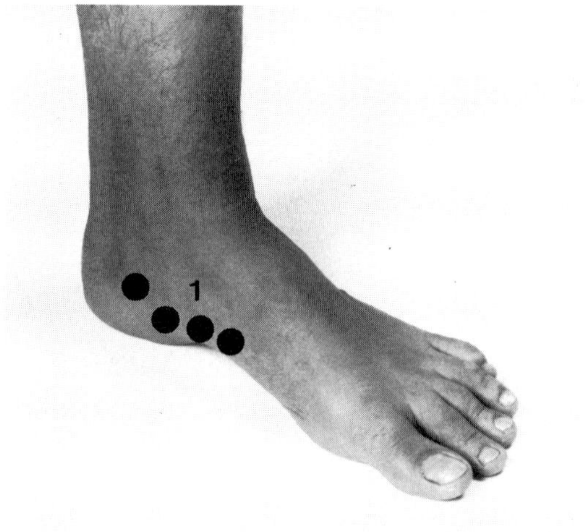


**Point 1**
(Reflex zone of the foot)
Located on the medial side of the heel bone. The points will react painfully to touch.

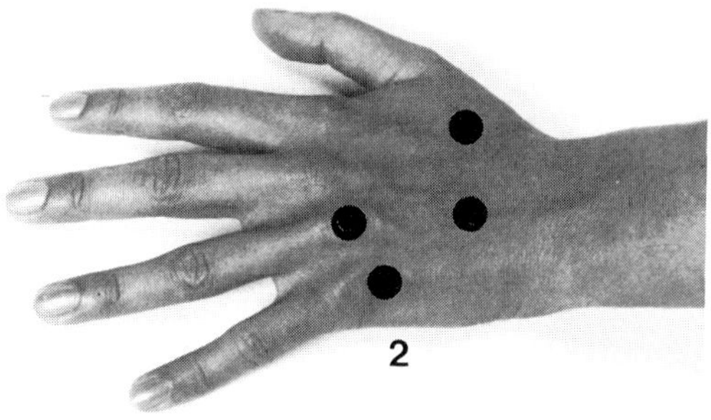


**Point 2**
(Reflex zones of the hand) - Back of hand
This combination consists of four points:
A) is located on the basal joint of the little finger;
B) lies on a line running from between the index and middle finger;
C) lies on a line running from between the ring and the little finger;
D) is located on the basal joint of the ring finger.

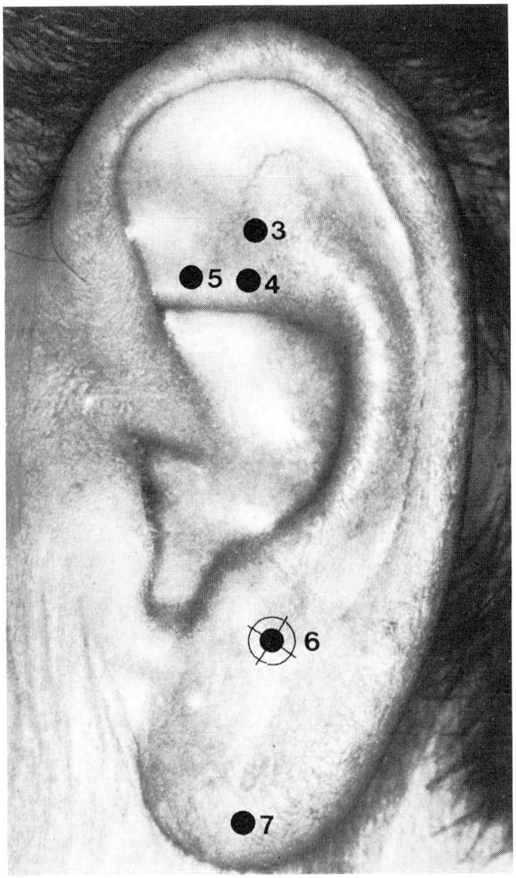


**Point 3** Ear point
**Point 4** Ear point
**Point 5** Ear point
**Point 6** Ear point
This point, which is indicated for the treatment of pain, is located on the inside of the lobe.
**Point 7** Ear point

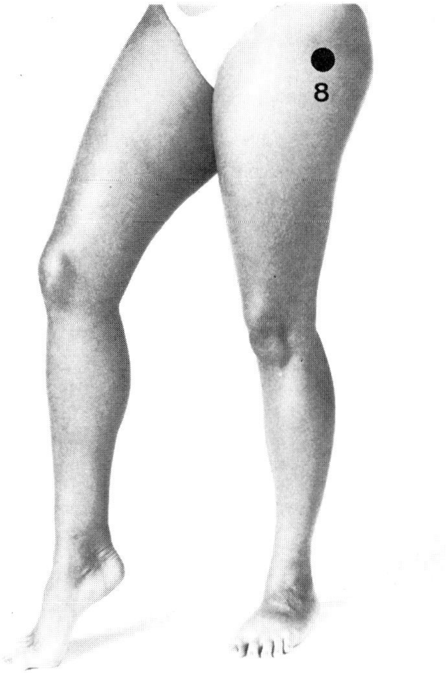


**Point 8**
(Gall bladder 30) Left and right
This point can be found on the outermost part of the hip joint.

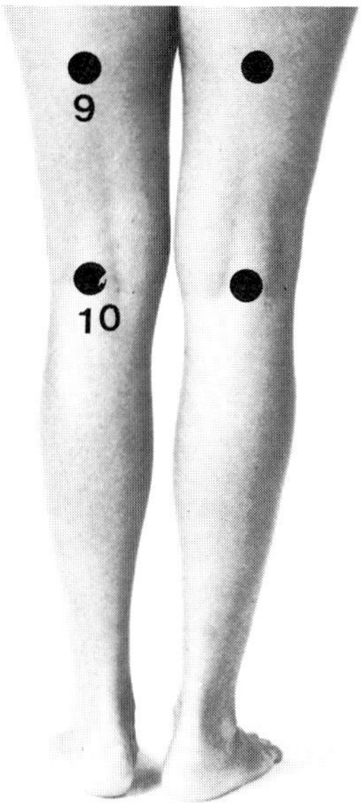


**Point 9**
(Bladder 51) Left and right
This point lies a handbreadth below the crease formed by the buttock.

**Point 10**
(Bladder 54) Left and right
Located in the middle of the hollow of the knee.

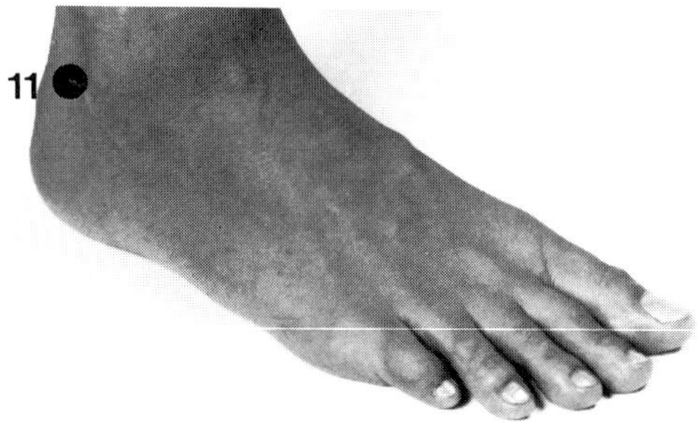


**Point 11**
(Bladder 60) Left and right

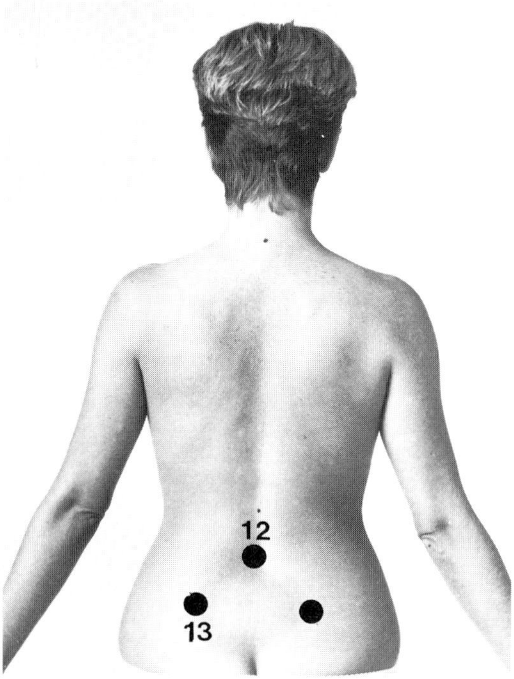


**Point 12**
(L5 - S1)
Located on the midline of the body, between the spinal process of the 5th lumbar vertebra and the sacrum.

**Point 13**
(Point of the pelvis)
Located in the middle of the iliac crest.

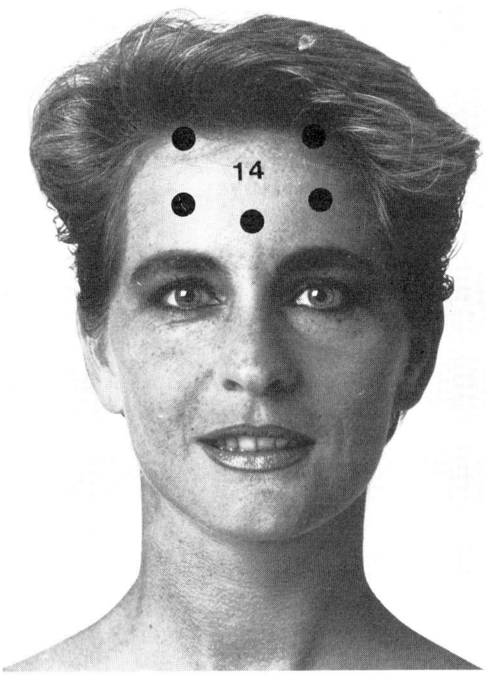


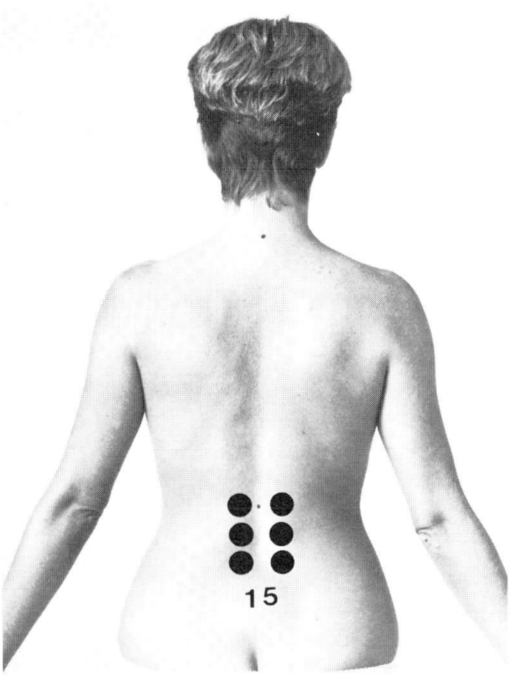


**Point 14**

A) (Thalamus point)

B) (Hypothalamus point)
Located on a line that leads up from the middle of the eye to the hairline.

C) (The limbic system)
This point is located 2 fingerbreadths above point B) and 1 fingerbreadth below the hair line.

**Point 15** (paravertebral)
These points are located 1 fingerbreadth to the left and right of the middle of the spine.

In the same way as sciatica, neural pain running down from the shoulder girdle into the arms and fingers can be excrutiating, long-lasting and nerve-wracking. It is generally caused in the cervical spine and the upper thoracic spine, but foci and disturbances of the gastrointestinal tract and the kidneys can also be responsible for this complaint. The points given here have all proved their worth, but, as in the case of sciatica again, a certain amount of patience will be necessary. Generally speaking, the impulses transmitted by the acu-impulsor will bring about a release of blocked or congested energy and thus relieve the pain involved. Start treatment on the pain-free side of the body and apply ten impulses per point.

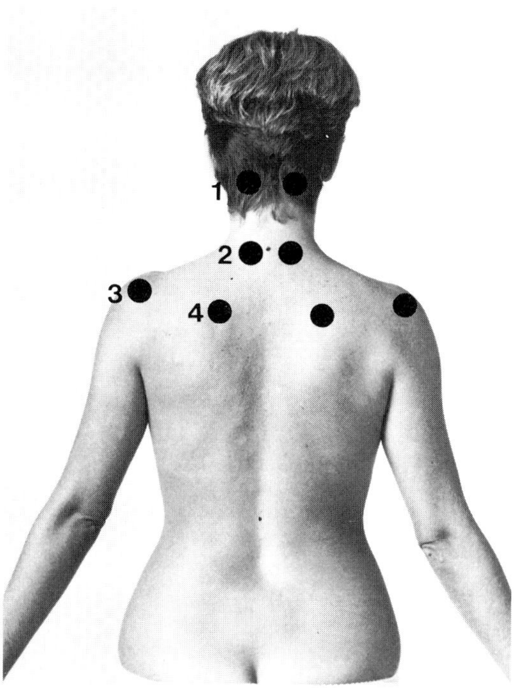


**Point 1**
(1st cervical vertebra)
Located between the 1st cervical vertebra and the skull, 1 fingerbreadth to the right and left of the midline of the body.

**Point 2**
(C 7) Left and right
Located at the most prominent protuberance of the cervical spine, approx. 1 fingerbreadth to the right and left of the spine.

**Point 3**
(L.I. 15) Left and right
Positioned at the outermost corner of the shoulder, in the little crease that forms when the arm is lifted.

**Point 4**
Located on the medial tip of the shoulder blade.

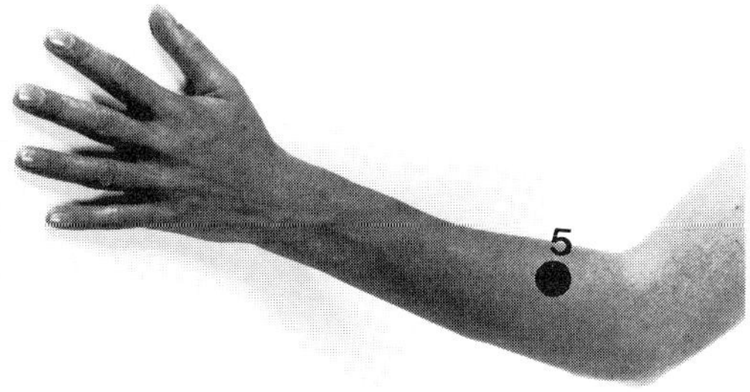


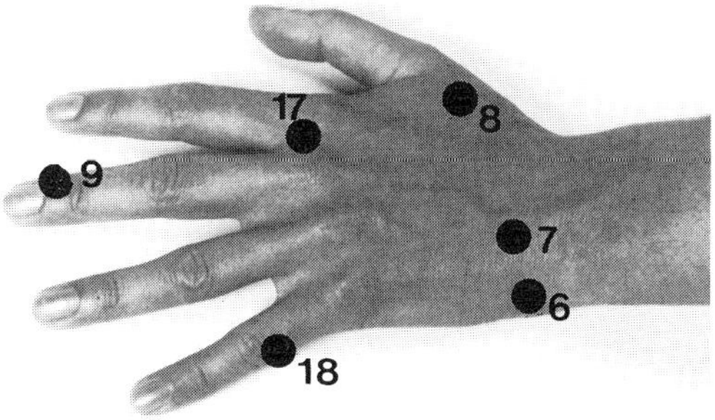


**Point 5**
(L. I. 10) Left and right
Located on the outer part of the outstretched arm, approx. 2 fingerbreadths away from the elbow crease.
This point is very painful and therefore easy to find.

**Point 6**
(S.I. 4) Left and right
Located on the outer edge of the hand, where a little gap can be felt in the joints.

**Point 7**
(T.H. 4) Left and right
Located in the fold of the wrist on a line leading from between the ring and little finger.

**Point 8**
(L.I. 4) Left and right
Located in the angle formed by the metacarpal bones of the thumb and index finger.

**Point 9**
(C. 9)
Located on the medial side of the distal phalanx of the 2nd finger, 2 mm away from the angle of the nail bed.

**Points 17 + 18**
(Reflex zones of the hand)
Point 17 is located on the lateral side of the basal joint of the index finger.
Point 18 is located on the lateral side of the metatarsal joint of the little finger.

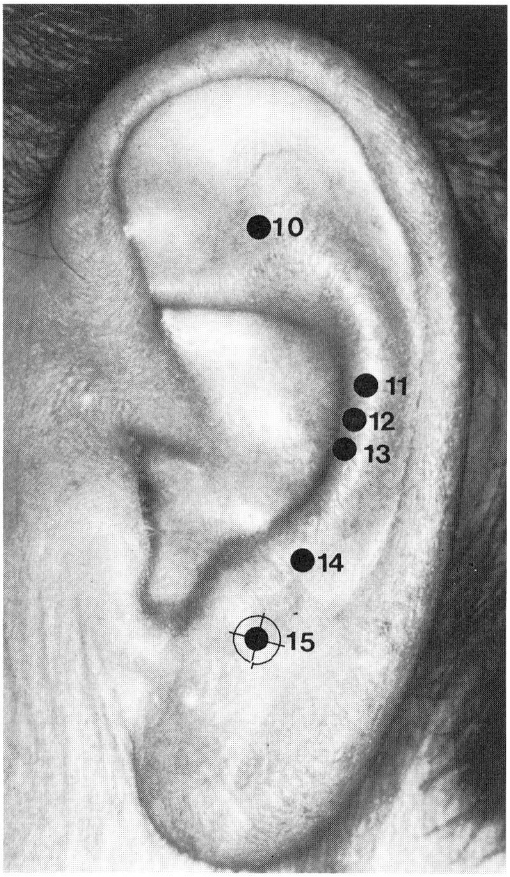


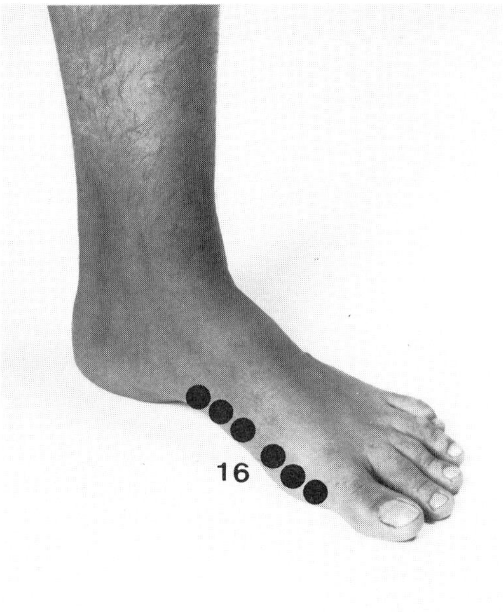


**Point 16**
(Reflex zone of the foot)
This collection of points starts at the basal joint of the big toe and runs along the arch of the foot.

**Point 10** Ear point
**Point 11** Ear point
**Point 12** Ear point
**Point 13** Ear point
**Point 14** Ear point
**Point 15** Ear point

# Complaints of the Joints

1. Activating the Metabolism
2. Rheumatic Complaints of the Joints
3. Complaints of the Joints in Conjunction with Gout
4. Arthrosis
5. Tennis Elbow
6. Four Point Joint Treatment
7. General, Less Severe Complaints of the Joints
8. Acute Lumbago

Complaints of the joints are among the most common syndromes encountered. The number of patients seeking relief of these complaints from conventional doctors and practitioners of natural therapeutics are legion.

We differentiate here between rheumatic-inflammatory processes, inflammations of the joints caused by gout, arthritis and arthrosis. All these complaints, however, have one common denominator, namely the fact that they are caused by altered metabolic functioning and also by foci of all kinds, which are particularly significant in this context. A weak immune system is also a potential cause.
As a matter of principle the patient as a whole must be regarded and not just the affected joints. Particularly with complaints of this type the interaction of many factors in the organism must always be taken into consideration. The first step consists of examining the patient's diet and food habits. In most cases there will be an excessive intake of meat or sweet foods, or an overindulgence in smoking and alcoholic beverages. When the body is no longer able to compensate the negative effects of the above mentioned factors, a general toxic situation arises. Rheumatism and complaints of the joints should always be treated by a physician or licensed health practitioner.

Nevertheless, it is particularly necessary for patients to learn to help themselves in overcoming pain and their restricted range of movement. A radical change to a balanced, healthy diet eliminating sugar and alcohol is an absolute necessity. Measures which patients can carry out at home include medicinal baths and packs, as well as therapeutic exercises and the application of liniments. The definition given by a well known German physician is particularly appropriate in this context: "Pain is the cry of the tissue for flowing energy". Therefore I began to integrate instructions for self-treatment into my therapy at an early stage. The simple manipulations with the acu-impulsor have proved highly effective here. The self-treatment carried out by the patient does not address itself primarily to the affected joint, but begins with a treatment of the lymphatic system in accordance with the complex nature of these syndromes. The initial treatment concentrates on the lymphatic system and the immune system and is carried daily over a two week period. The second phase consists of treating metabolism points which have a special affinity to the muscles and joints. This treatment is also carried out for a period of two weeks in daily alternation with lymph therapy. Specific combinations for the affected joints are applied after four weeks of these preliminary measures.

During the first four weeks it is important for the patient to adhere to a balanced and healthy diet and also to make sure that his or her liquid intake is sufficient (two liters of water per day). Practical experience has shown that the complaints often improve to a considerable degree during this period of time so that by the time the specific therapeutic combinations for the joints are applied, the organism already possesses improved capacity for regeneration. Treatment is carried out as follows:

1. 14 days of lymph treatment
2. 14 days of daily alteration between the treatment of the metabolism points and the !ymph therapy points.
3. Make the change to a balanced, healthy diet, and eliminate alcoholic beverages and sugar. Apply hot compresses to the liver and treat inflamed joints with cool compresses.

The affected joints can also be treated with individually prescribed herbal liniments.

4. After four weeks the following point combinations are integrated into the self-treatment program, whereby the lymph and metabolism combinations are still carried out once a week.

Your patience and perseverance will be rewarded with a reduction of pain and in many cases with a complete cure.

(Lymph treatment – see page 37)

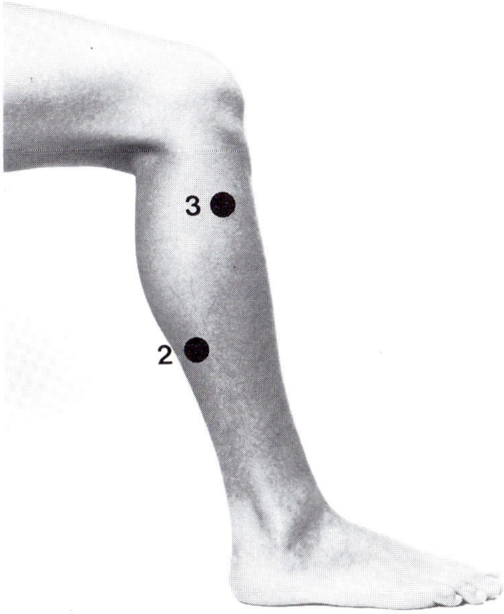


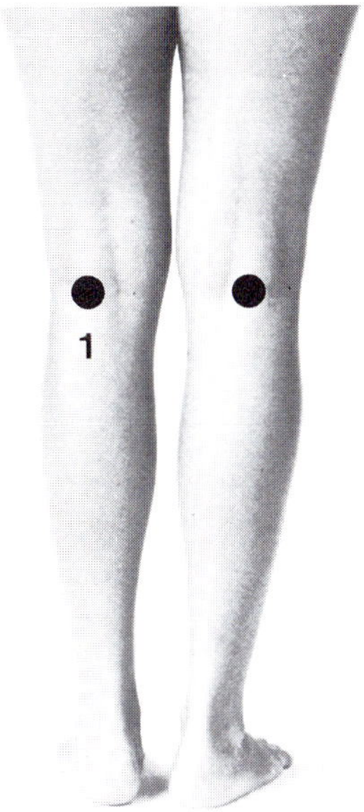


**Point 1**
(U.B. 54) Left and right
Located in the middle of the hollow of the knee.

**Point 2**
(U.B. 58) Left and right
Located on the lateral side of the calf.

**Point 3**
(St. 36) Left and right
This point is situated on the frontal surface of the leg, 3 fingerbreadths beneath the knee on the shin bone. Another way of locating this point is to place the palm of your hand on your kneecap. The point is situated at the tip of your middle finger.

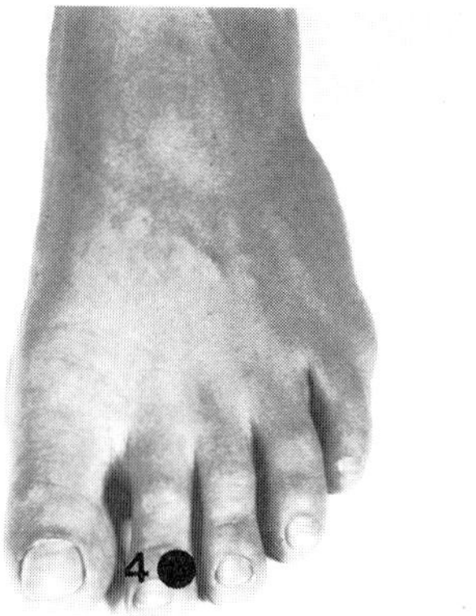


**Point 4**
(St. 45) Left and right
Located on the second toe approximately 2 mm at a diagonal from the lateral angle of the nailbed groove.

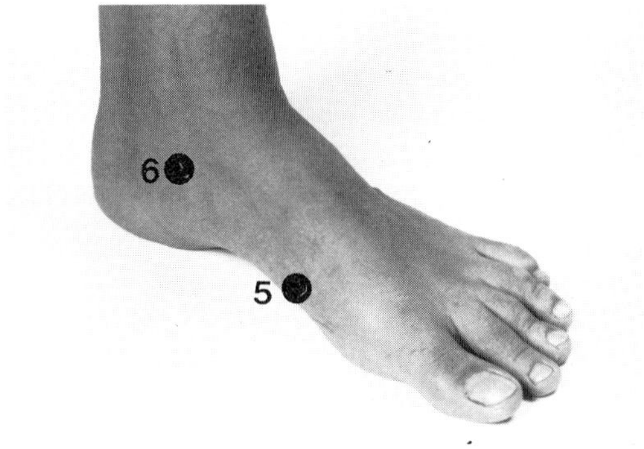


**Point 5**
(K. 2) Left and right
Located laterally at the midsection of the foot.

**Point 6**
(K. 6) Left and right
Located approximately 1 fingerbreadth away from the malleolus in the direction of the large toe.

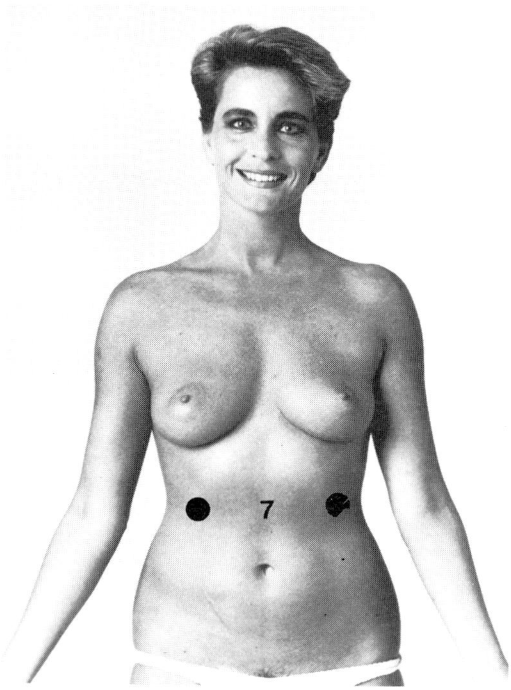


**Point 7**
(Liv. 13) Left and right
Located on the 11th rib, somewhat medially of its distal end.

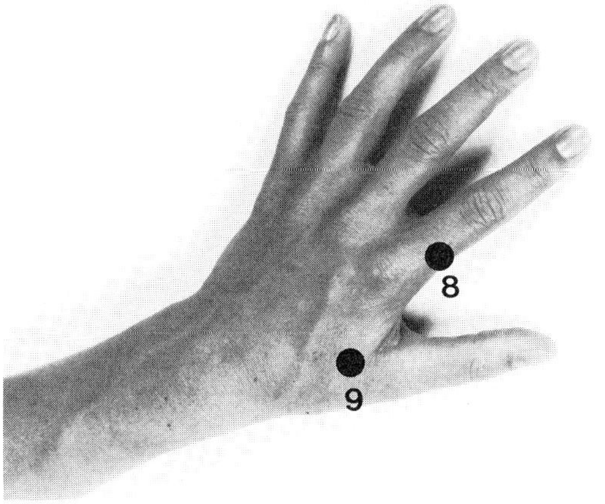


**Point 8**
(L.I. 2) Left and right
Located medially, approximately 1 fingerbreadth away from the metatarsal joint of the index finger.

**Point 9**
(L.I. 4) Left and right
Located medially on the index finger where the metacarpal bones of index finger and thumb meet.

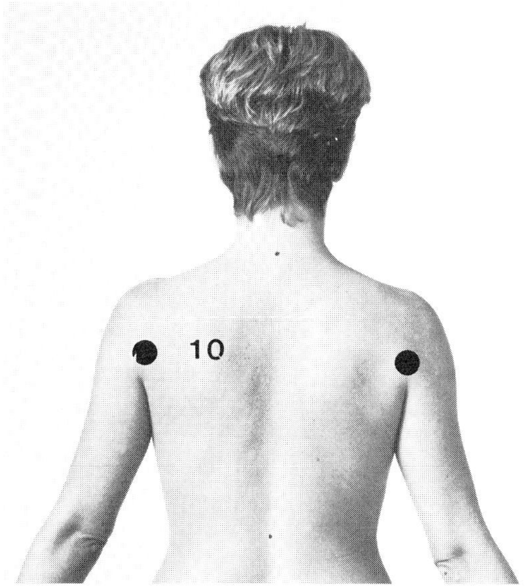


**Point 10**
(S.I. 9) Left and right
Located 2 fingerbreadths above the axillar fold.

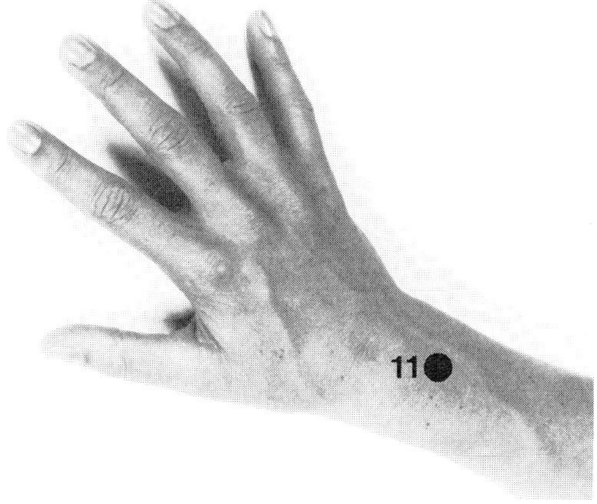


**Point 11**
(T.H. 5) Left and right
This point is situated approximately 2½ fingerbreadths above the fold of the wrist in the middle between ulna and radius.

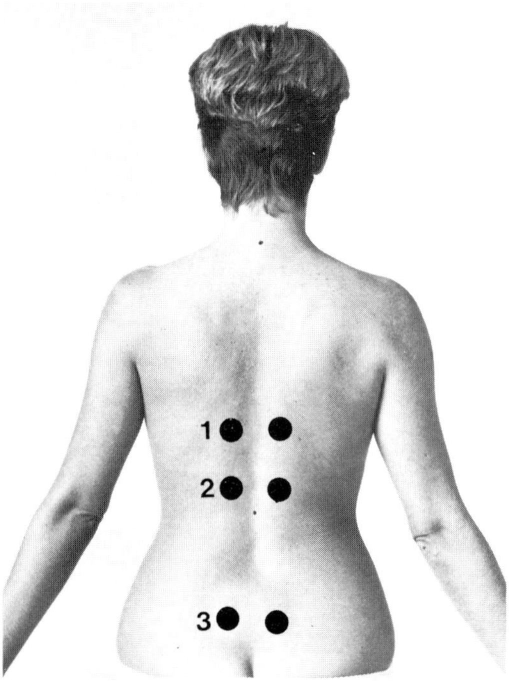


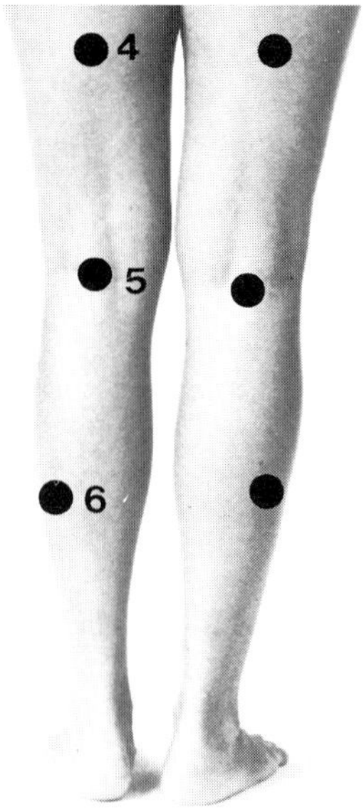


**Point 1**
(U.B. 17) Left and right
Located in the 7th intercostal space, 2 fingerbreadths from the midline of the body.

**Point 2**
(U.B. 21) Left and right
Situated in the 12 intercostal space, 2 fingerbreadths from the midline of the body.

**Point 3**
(U.B. 29) Left and right
Located on the same level as the 3rd sacral canal, approx. 3 fingerbreadths from the midline of the body.

**Point 4**
(U.B. 51) Left and right
Located 1 handbreadth beneath the fold formed by the gluteal muscle.

**Point 5**
(U.B. 54) Left and right
Lies in the middle of the hollow of the knee.

**Point 6**
(U.B. 58) Left and right
Located at the middle of the calf on the lateral surface.

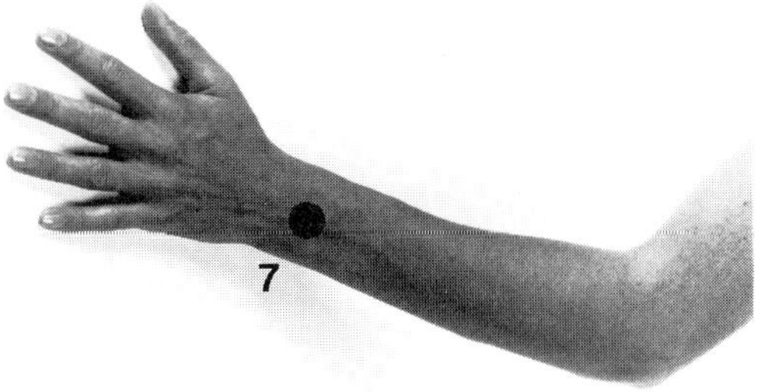


**Point 7**
(T.H. 5) Left and right
This point is located approximately 2 ½ finger-breadths above the fold of the wrist in the middle between ulna and radius.

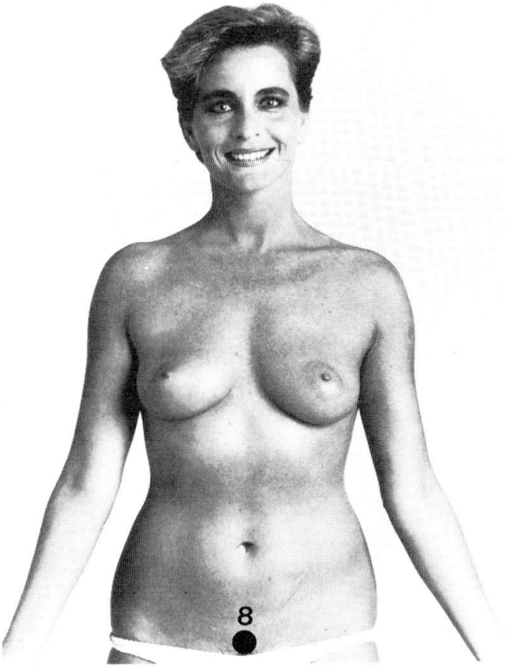


**Point 8**
(C.V. 3)
Located 2 fingerbreadths above the pubic bone in the midline of the body.

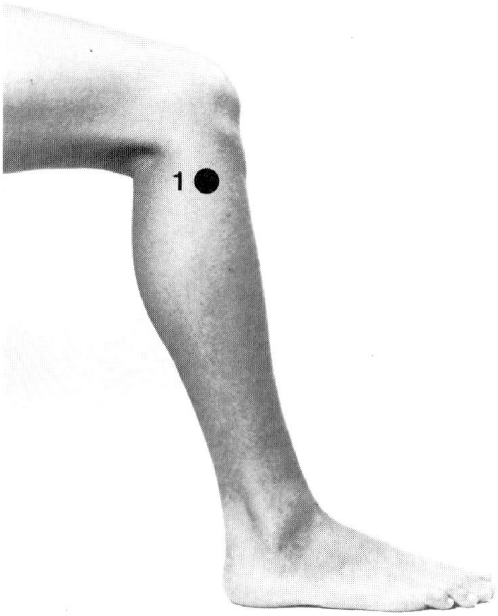


**Point 1**
(G.B. 34) Left and right
Located on the lateral surface of the lower leg, where a small hollow is formed when the knee is bent.

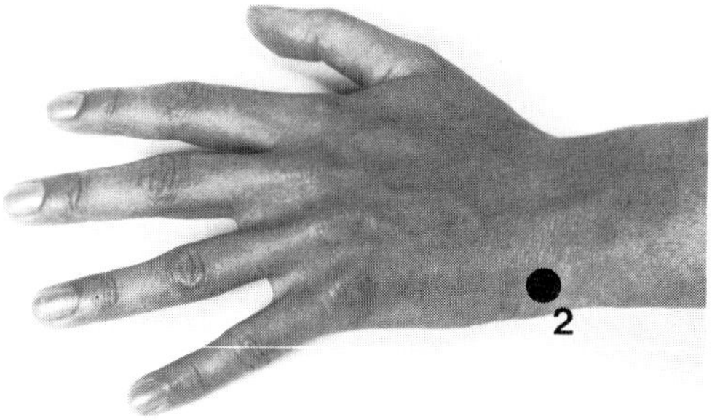


**Point 2**
(S.I. 4)
Located on the lateral margin of the hand where a small gap can be felt in the joint.

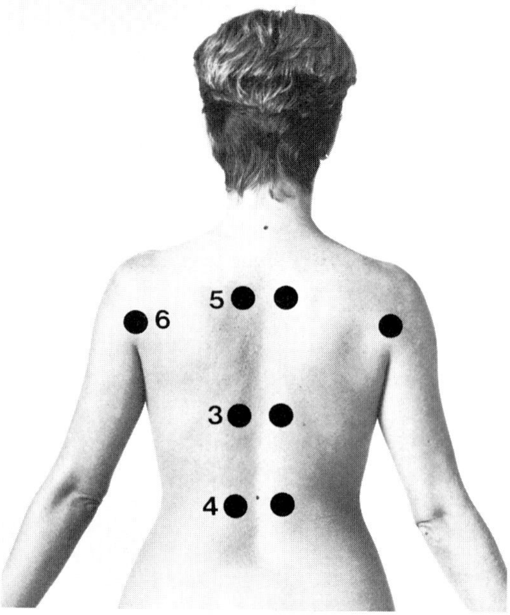


**Point 3**
(U.B. 18) Left and right
Located in the 9th intercostal space, 2 fingerbreadths away from the midline of the body.

**Point 4**
(U.B. 23) Left and right
Located between the 2nd and 3rd lumbar vertebra, 2 fingerbreadths away from the midline of the body.

**Point 5**
(U.B. 13) Left and right
Located in the 3rd intercostal space, 2 fingerbreadths away from the midline of the body.

**Point 6**
(S.I. 9) Left and right
Situated two fingerbreadths above the axillar fold.

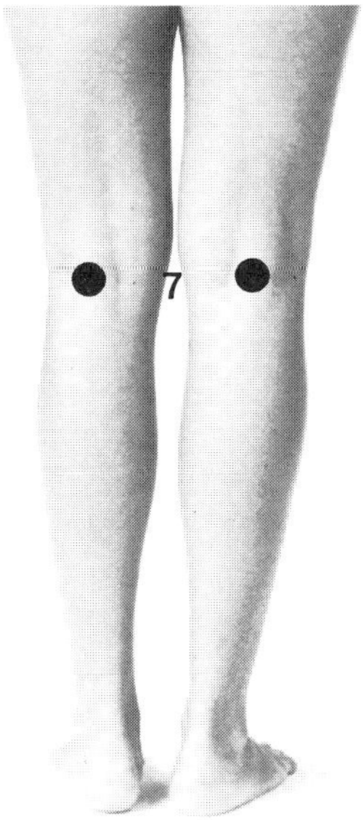


**Point 7**
(U.B. 54) Left and right
Located in the middle of the hollow of the knee.

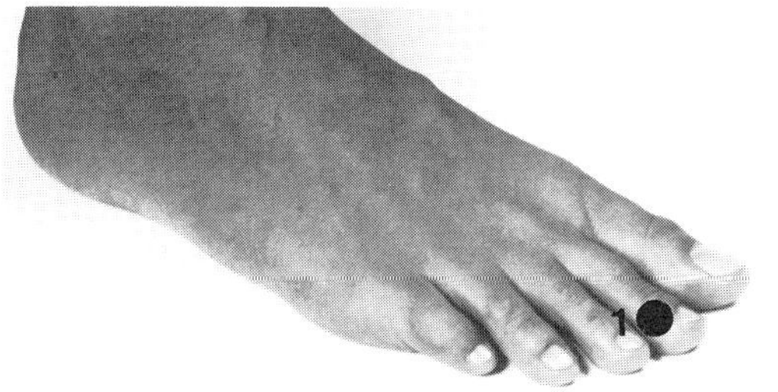


**Point 1**
(St. 45) Left and right
This point is situated on the lateral surface of the second toe, approx. 2 mm diagonally offset from the angle of the nailbed groove.

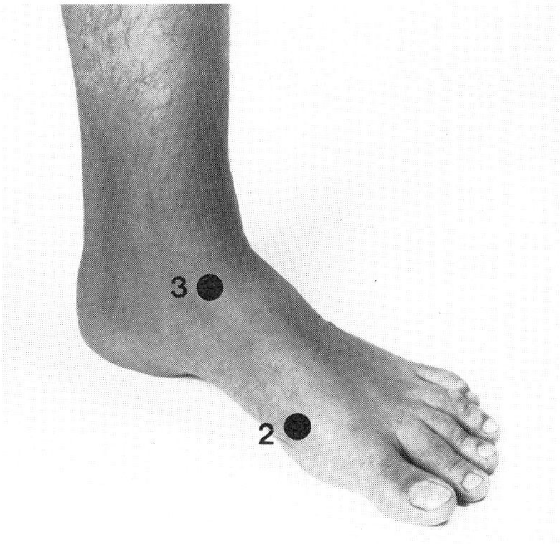


**Point 2**
(P. 3) Left and right
Located on the medial margin of the foot, approx. 1 fingerbreadth away from the basal joint of the large toe.

**Point 3**
(P. 5) Left and right
Located on the medial surface of the back of the foot, approx. 2 fingerbreadths below the ankle joint.

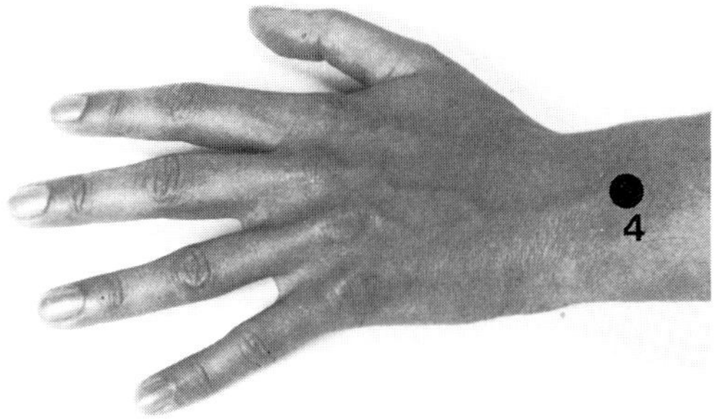


**Point 4**
(T.H. 5) Left and right
Located approx. 2½ fingerbreadths above the fold of the wrist in the middle between ulna and radius.

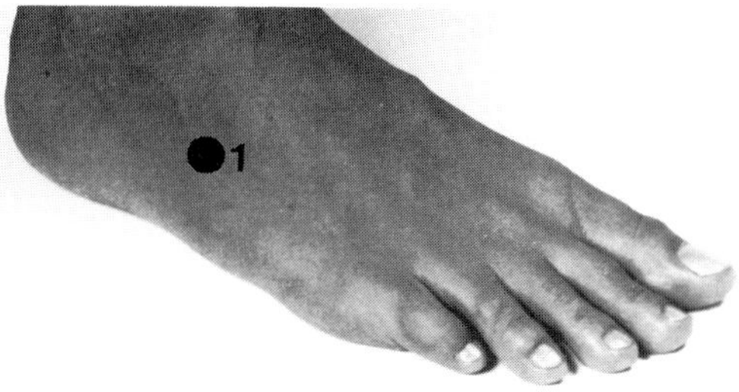


**Point 1**
(G.B. 41) Left and right
Lies on the back of the foot between the metatarsal bones of the 4th and 5th toe at their proximal ends.

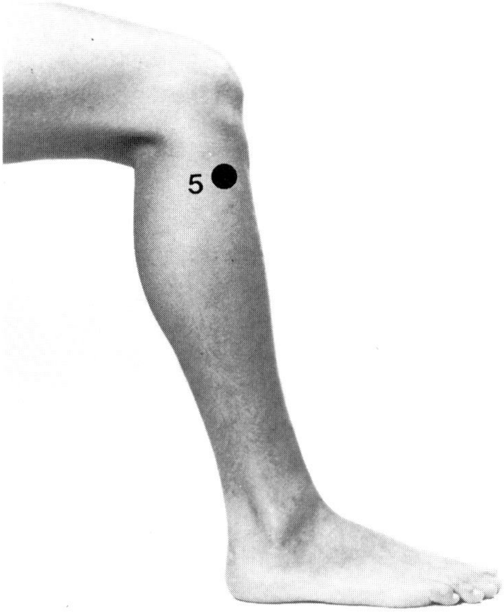


**Point 5**
(St. 36) left and right
This point is situated on the frontal surface of the leg, 3 fingerbreadths beneath the knee on the shin bone. Another way of locating this point is to place the palm of your hand on your kneecap. The point is situated at the tip of your middle finger.

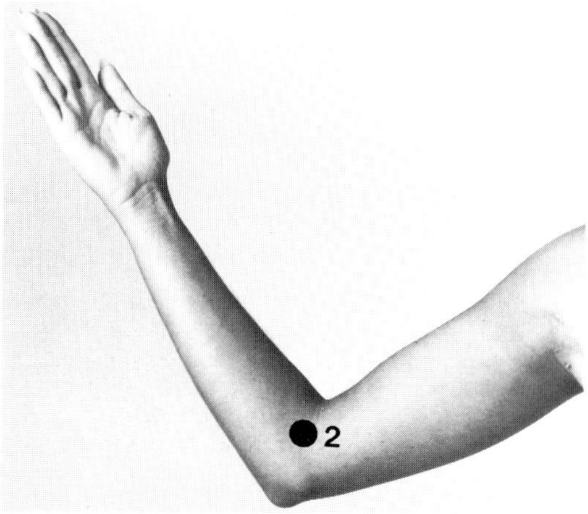


**Point 2**
(H. 2) Left and right
Located at the lateral end of the elbow fold when the lower arm is bent.

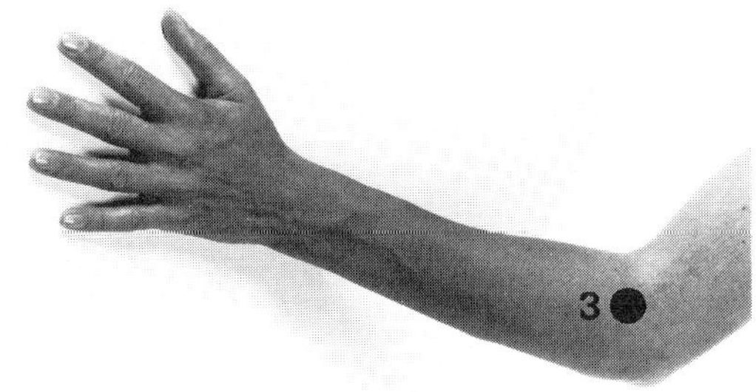


**Point 3**
(S.I. 11) Left and right
Lies at the lateral end of the external elbow fold.

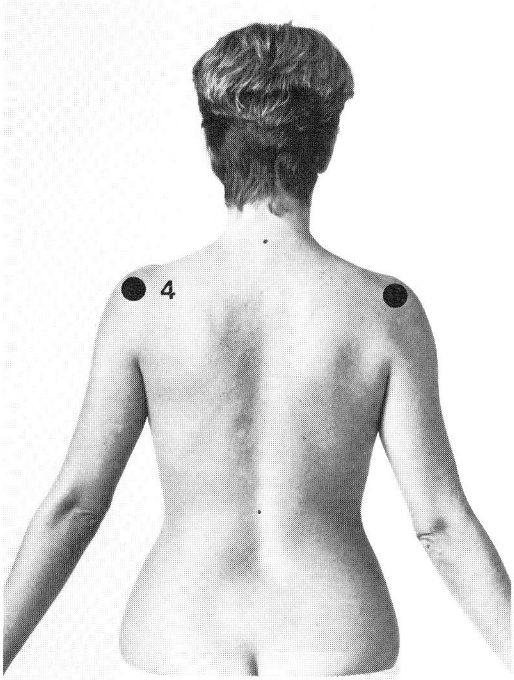


**Point 4**
(S.I. 15) Left and right
Situated at the external margin of the shoulder, in the middle of a small hollow produced by raising the arm to a horizontal position.

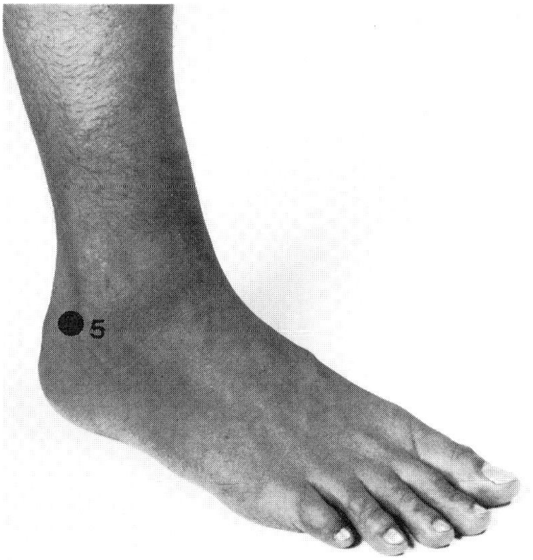


**Point 5**
(U.B. 60) Left and right
Positioned on the lateral surface of the foot between the malleolus and the achilles tendon.

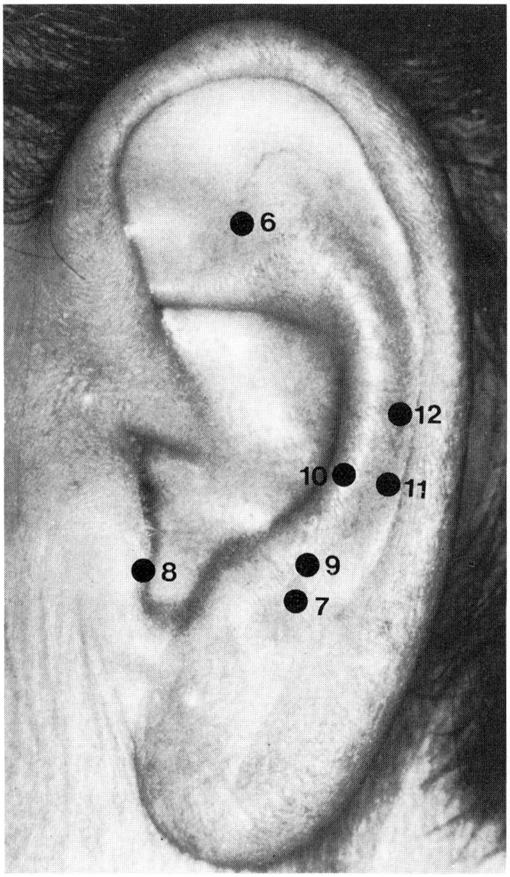


**Point 6:** Ear point
**Point 7:** Ear point
**Point 8:** Ear point
**Point 9:** Ear point
**Point 10:** Ear point
**Point 11:** Ear point
**Point 12:** Ear point

These points are especially valuable for persons who tend to strain one of their arms in particularly, such as tennis players. In such cases, this treatment can be carried out as prophylactic measure.

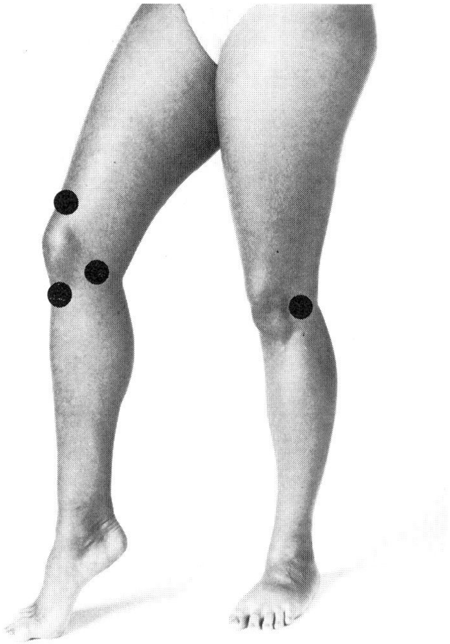

I discovered the following new combination of points for degenerative complaints of the joints (absence of inflammation) during the course of my work with Colorpuncture. These points are arranged in the form of a rhombus, whereby in all cases only one of the four will be found to be painful. Our illustration shows the knee joint as an example. Locate the points and mark the painful ones. The three less painful points are treated first by stimulating them ten times each and repeating this measure twice at three minute intervals. In conclusion, the painful point is given ten impulses. This arthrosis treatment can be repeated daily until the complaints are ameliorated. As the condition improves, the intervals between individual treatments should be increased.

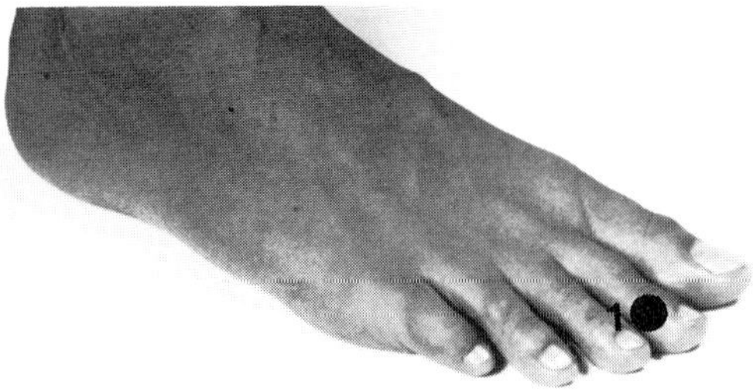


**Point 1**
(St. 45) Left and right
This point is situated on the lateral surface of the second toe, approx. 2 mm diagonally offset from the angle of the nailbed groove.

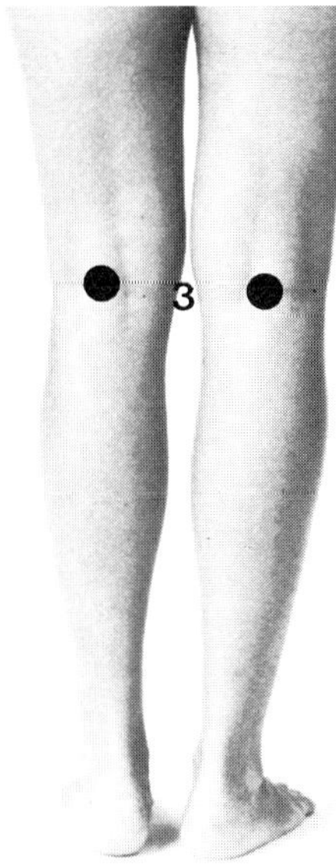


**Point 3**
(U.B. 54) Left and right
Lies in the middle of the hollow of the knee.

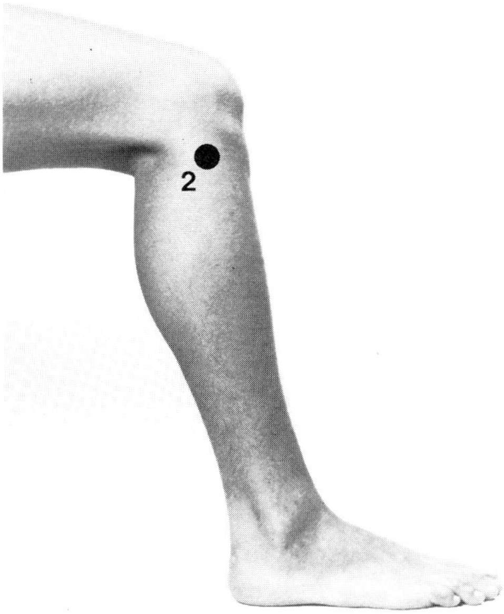


**Point 2**
(G.B. 34) Left and right
Located on the lateral surface of the lower leg, where a small hollow is formed when the knee is bent.

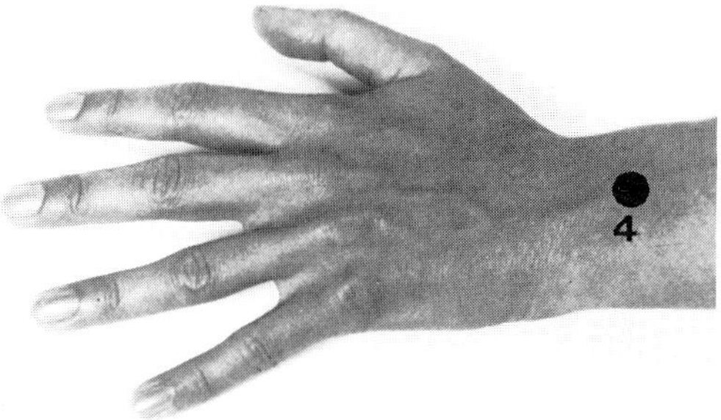


**Point 4**
(T.H. 5) Left and right
Located approx. 2½ fingerbreadths above the fold of the wrist in the middle between ulna and radius.

Those of us who have experienced acute lumbago will certainly not forget the incident so quickly. Whatever the cause may have been - lifting or straining, lying in the wrong position or taking cold - the acu-impulsor treatment of the following points is an effective initial self-help measure. Assuming the position shown in the drawing on page 94 has proved helpful in many cases. Applying warmth to the affected parts, perhaps in the manner of our grandparents with a pack of hot boiled potatoes, may bring additional relief.

The following points are for cases of acute pain:

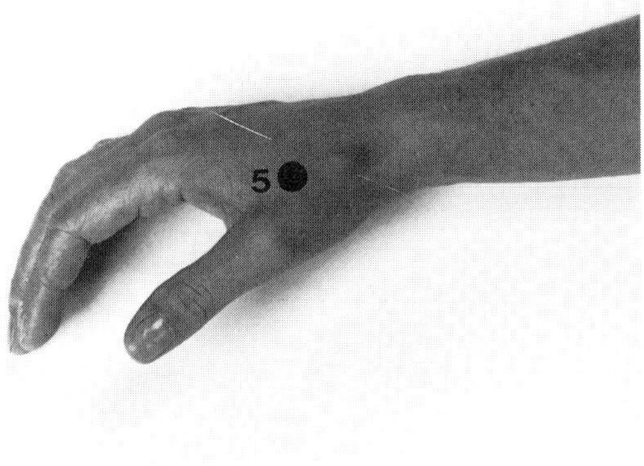


**Point 5**
(L.I. 4) Left and right
Located on the medial surface of the index finger where the metacarpal bones of the index finger and thumb meet.

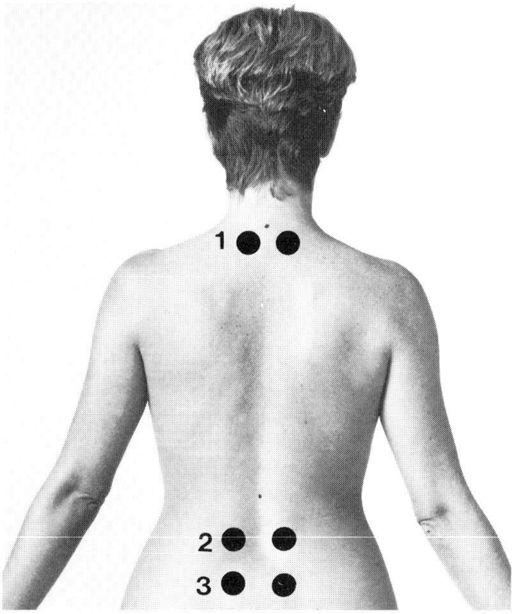


**Point 1**
(U.B. 11) Left and right
Located in the 1st intercostal space, 2 fingerbreadths away from the midline of the body.

**Point 2**
(U.B. 25) Left and right
Situated 2 fingerbreadths away from the midline of the body between the 4th and the 5th lumbar vertebra.
**Point 3**
(U.B. 31) Left and right
Located on the medial side of the 1st sacral canal.

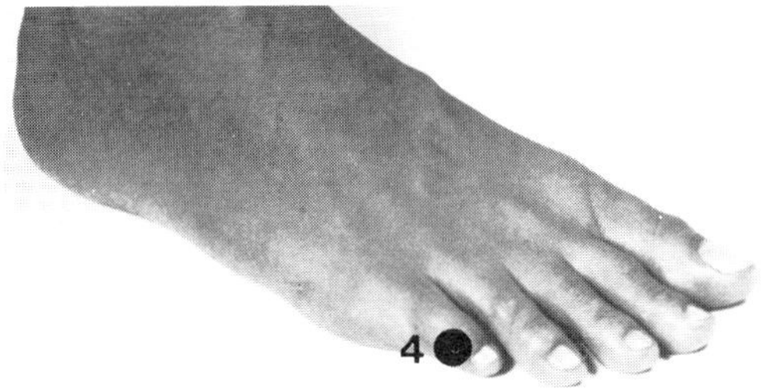


**Point 4**
(U.B. 67) Left and right
Located on the lateral nail bed groove of the small toe, approx. 2 mm away from the angle of the nail bed.

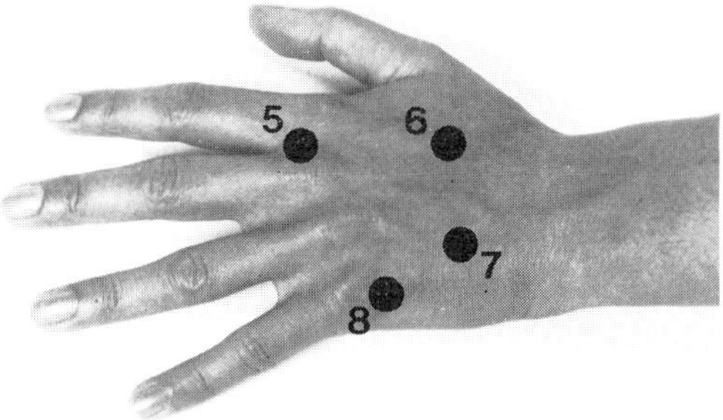


**Point 5** (Web margin) Left and right
Situated on the web margin between the index and middle finger.
**Point 6 + 7**
These points are located on the back of the hand on a line drawn between the distal ends of the 1st and 3rd metacarpals.
**Point 8** This point is situated on the basal joint of the small finger.

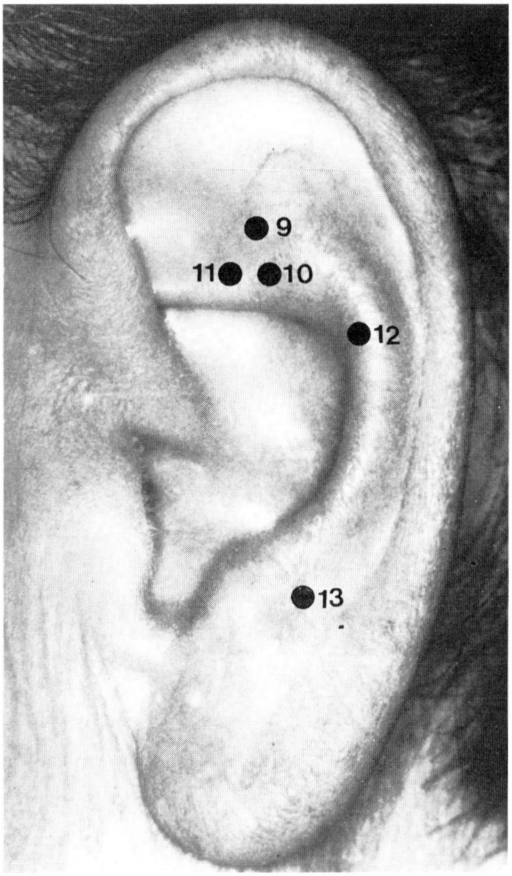


**Point 9:** Ear point
**Point 10:** Ear point
**Point 11:** Ear point
**Point 12:** Ear point
**Point 13:** Ear point

Ten impulses per point are applied in the above specified sequence and this treatment is repeated 3 to 4 times. If an intervertebral disc is affected and conservative treatment has been opted for, the following points are added:

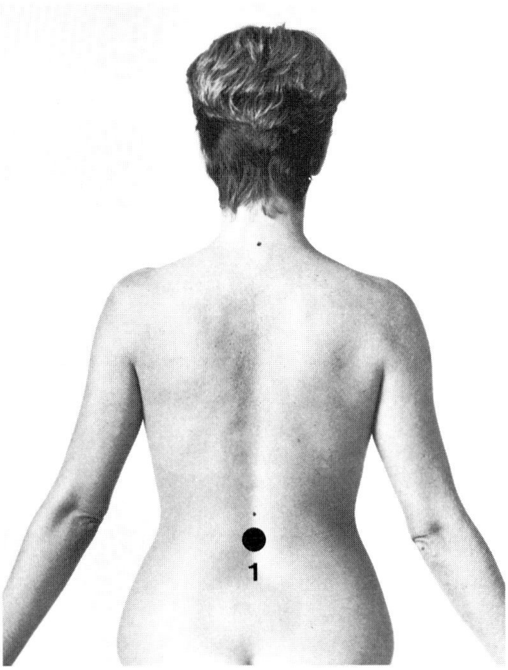


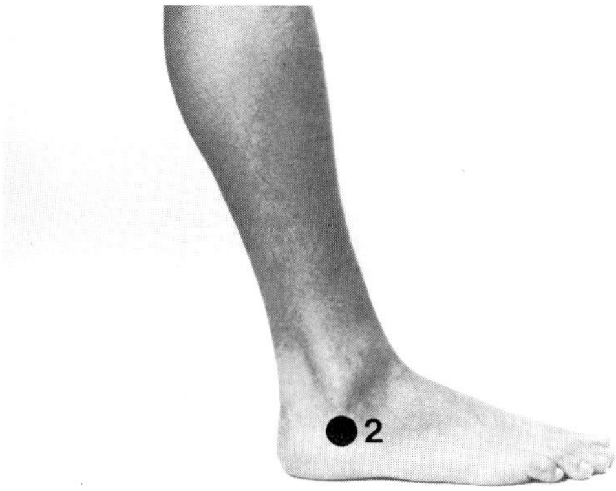


**Point 2**
(U.B. 62) Left and right
This point is located 2 fingerbreadths beneath the lateral malleolus.

**Point 1**
(G.V. 4)
Situated on the spinal process of the 2nd lumbar vertebra.

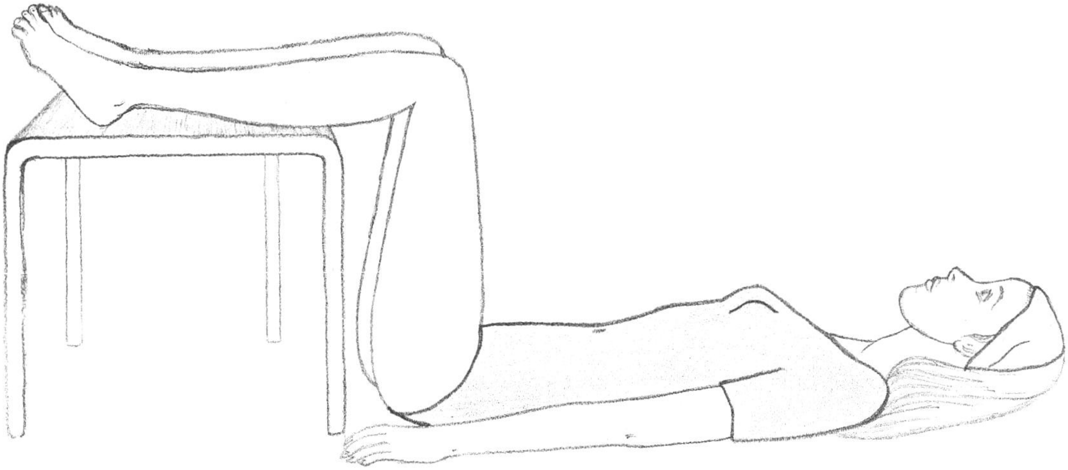

Position for acute lumbago

The preceding pages have concentrated on the treatment of particularly common diseases and types of pain with the acu-impulsor.

The second section of this book focuses on a further series of common complaints and syndromes which can be successfully treated with the acu-impulsor. Be sure to follow the instructions which specify the sequence of points and the repetition of treatment. At the same time, however, we should also be aware of the fact that there is more to staying healthy than regulating the organism's energetic potential. Health depends on many other factors. Some can be favorably affected by the acu-impulsor, while others are determined entirely by the person involved. Diet and food habits, exaggerated egotism and stress-causing behavioral patterns must be dealt with effectively. Without the individual's will to change, even the best possible therapy is doomed to failure. Therefore, it is necessary to be able to imagine oneself in a state of health and well-being. Happiness, contentment and a certain humility toward one's fellow men should be goals we all seek to attain. Regardless of one's faith or beliefs, it is well for the individual to reflect on the creation and on origin of man. In the endeavour to lead a life of harmony and overcome aggression and prejudice, we should always bear in mind that in the end we are indeed the result of our thoughts, and that negative thinking over a long period of time can quite literally destroy a person.

It is not my intention to discourse on the meaning of life or ethics, for the topic of this book is the regulation and balancing of the energetic potential within the organism. However, just like matter, the energy system within the body is without genuine substance unless awakened to life by the immaterial information which makes our existence possible, wherever it may stem from. The question as to where this information originates may never be answered. I believe it is an inherent part of the energy system which is transmitted to the individual when he or she comes into being, and that functional disturbances and disease are – in theory – impossible.
A Chinese master was once asked by his disciple: "What is disease?". I would like to conclude the first section of this book with the master's answer:

"Disease is a thought."

The second part of the book is concerned with a number of common diseases and syndromes, which are mainly of chronic nature. In most cases, the conventional allopathic treatment of these disorders demands a great amount of medication.

I have decided to omit lengthy descriptions of the individual syndromes and concentrate on treatment with the acu-impulsor instead.

It is important to localize the indicated points and zones as accurately as possible, which should pose no great difficulties since they will be found to be sensitive to pressure. Use the rod which has been provided along with the acu-impulsor to help sense the indicated points and zones and treat those found most sensitive.

Treat each point with ten impulses each in accordance with the given sequences and always begin on the left-hand side. Carry out treatment as regularly as possible. As a general rule manifest symptoms and complaints are treated once or even twice daily. Once an improvement has set in, treatment should be carried out at greater intervals. Once symptoms have disappeared, keep using the energy balancing combinations in order to maintain the pain-free or balanced condition.

Now is the best time to start to improve your health and begin a better life!

# Nervous Complaints

1. Alternating Moods – Stage Fright
2. Anxiety
3. Depression
4. Sensation as of a Lump in the Throat
5. General Arteriosclerosis
6. Dizziness
7. Bed-Wetting
8. Developmental Disturbances in Children

Television and environmental pollution, the stress of everyday life and the rat race in general place a great strain on the human psyche these days. Therefore, it is not amazing that many people suffer from nervous complaints. Whether these consist of simple upsets or serious forms of loss of psychological control, the person involved is affected to the extent that he feels that life isn't worth living any more.
Restlessness, anxiety and even depression are also found in children and are to be taken seriously, especially in view of the damage these can cause to whole families.

Although it is often concealed or disguised, the principle of "an eye for an eye and a tooth for a tooth" dominates in our performance-oriented society. Those unable to fulfill society's expectations fall by the wayside, as evidenced by the many broken families and addicts of all kinds.
The distress thus caused makes life a farce. People should be able to live in happiness and harmony with their situation and surroundings. But what is the case if the situation and surroundings are not in harmony with the person? Resignation to this state amounts to loss of life, for it leads into the bottomless pit of anxiety, depression and destitution.
Many people are not thick-skinned. Yet, if they would they not let themselves be pushed into the confinements of a regulated form of life, they would be the happiest of people. Being sensitive and capable of feeling, they are to be envied, for they do not have to trample through life without expending a thought on the damage done. Instead, they are able to rely on their feelings. Such people must take care, however, not to be engulfed by the world around them. They can do so by not giving a chance to anxiety and restlessness and by nipping changes in mood in the bud. The weakness of their psychological makeup is not a handicap, but a gift, yet all the same, they should try to balance out their system once in a while with the acu-impulsor. Of course, the acu-impulsor will not turn a sensitive soul into a calculating and coldhearted person, but it will regulate an unbalanced flow of energy and the resulting misguided information. This will not only contribute to a durable state of harmony but will also help those affected by nervous complaints to cope with circumstances in a better way. Since they will now see things with different eyes, they will react accordingly and thus grow in inward strength.

I am of the opinion that nervous complaints are inseparably linked with the hormonal functions of the body. Many years of research with the Kirlian effect have shown me that there is a connection between the psyche and the endocrine system of the body.

For this reason, it would be inconceivable to treat nervous complaints in my practice without treating the endocrine system, for the one determines the other. As in the case of the hen and the egg, it would be useless to ask which one came first, however. In this respect, we simply have to think of how women react to the change of life or children to puberty. Both have to do with changes in the hormone house-hold and both involve changes in mood and temperament.

People in need of acu-impulsor treatment for these kinds of complaints should also carry out some other kind of therapy, such as autogenous training. Another possibility is meditating to the control exercises as part of my color-tone-therapy. There are many possibilities, and treatment with the acu-impulsor is simply one of them. However, it is one which is capable of regulating the flow of energy, thus ensuring a contented and harmonious approach to life.

If you wish to treat yourself for the abovementioned disorders, you should start out with the control exercises in the energy-balancing program.
Carry them out for once a day for 8 days and repeat them three times. Then you can continue on a daily basis with the following exercises, depending on case.
As usual, the better you feel and become, the less often you will need treatment. Remember, however, that you will also have to change your complete way of life. Make sure you get enough movement. Movement and correct breathing are just as important as meditation. And don't forget to start enjoying life again. It isn't easy, but if you follow the path of joy, you will get your reward – a peaceful and harmonious life led in happiness and absence of fear.

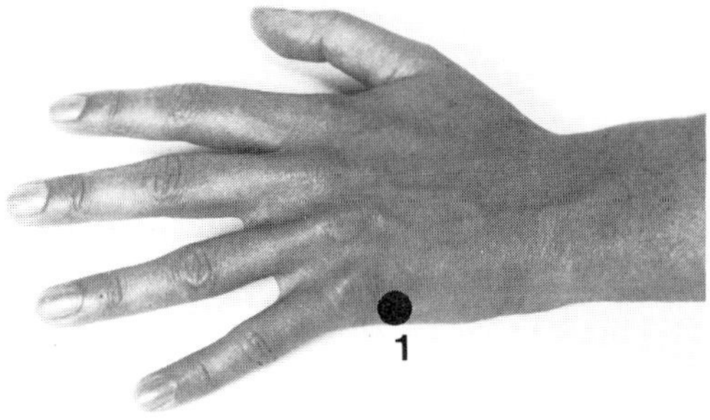


**Point 1**
(S.I. 3) Left and right
Located on the lateral side of the hand at the end of the large fold that is formed when the hand is clenched into a fist.

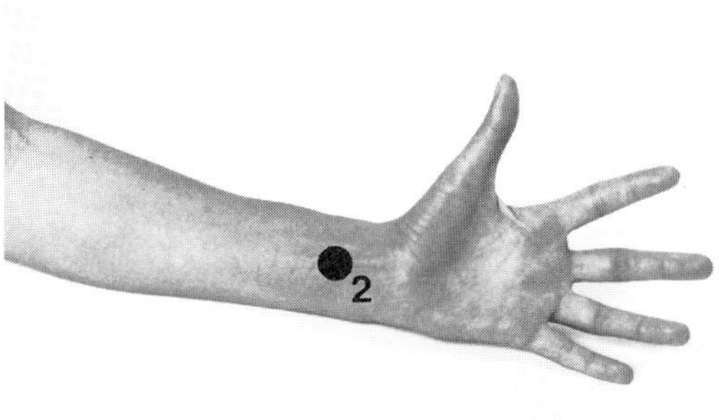


**Point 2**
(C. 6) Left and right
Located on the medial side of the forearm, 3 fingerbreadths above the fold of the wrist.

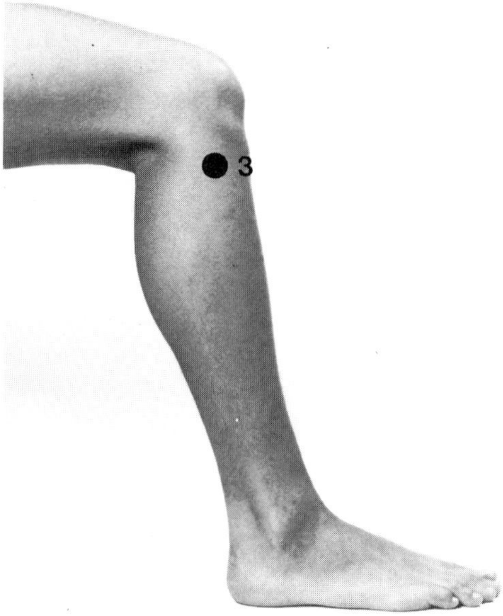


**Point 3**
(G.B. 34) Left and right
This point is located on the lateral side of the leg in the little hollow formed by bending the knee.

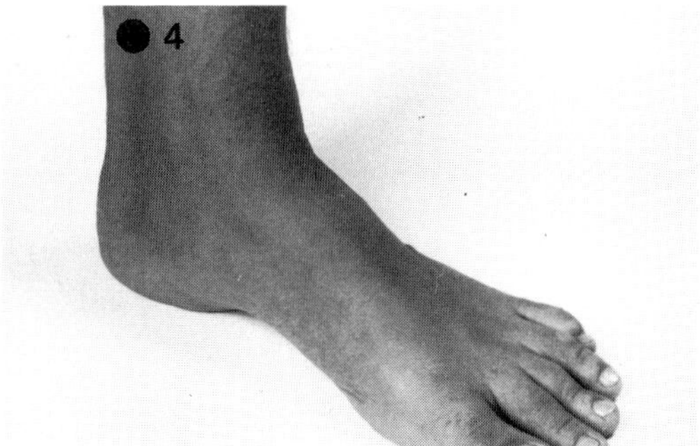


**Point 4**
(K. 7) Left and right
Draw an imaginary line leading 2 fingerbreadths up from the middle of the medial ankle. The point is located approx. 1 fingerbreadth away, towards the back of the leg.

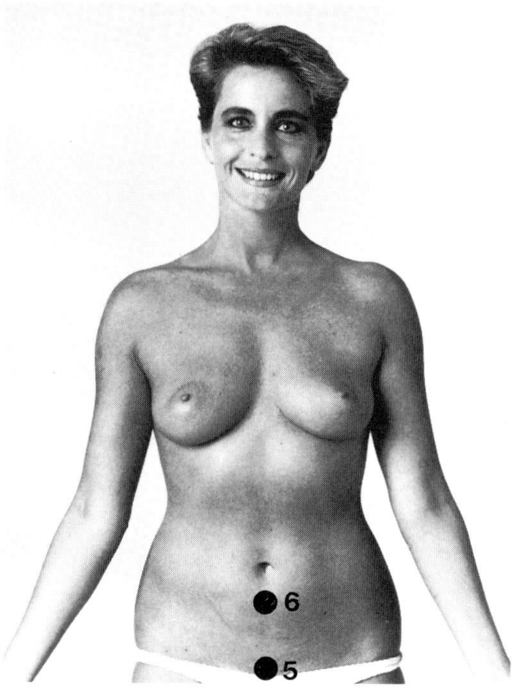


**Point 5**
(C.V. 3)
Located 2 fingerbreadths exactly above the middle of the pubic bone.

**Point 6**
(C.V. 6)
Located approx. 2 fingerbreadths below the navel.

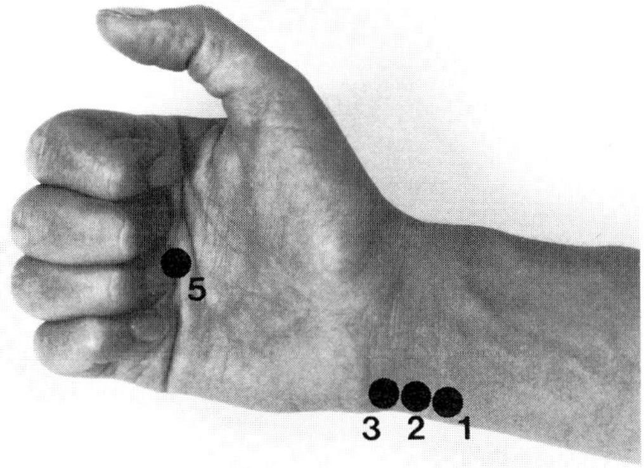


**Point 1**
(H. 5) Left and right
Located on the medial side of the forearm, 1 fingerbreadth above the line of the wrist.

**Point 2**
(H. 6 ) Left and right
Located ½ fingerbreadth above the line of the wrist on the medial side of the forearm.

**Point 3**
(H. 7) Left and right
Located on the 1st fold of the wrist.

**Point 5**
(C. 8) Left and right
The point is located between the tips of the middle and ring fingers when the hand is clenched into a fist.

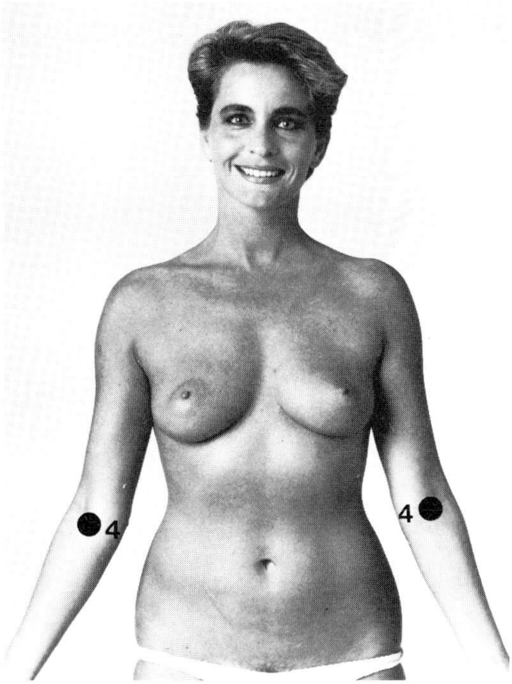


**Point 4**
(C. 3) Left and right
This point is located in the elbow on the little-finger-side of the vein of the musculus biceps.

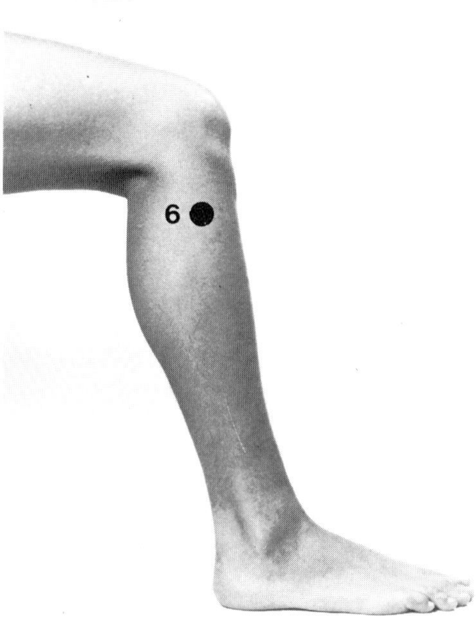


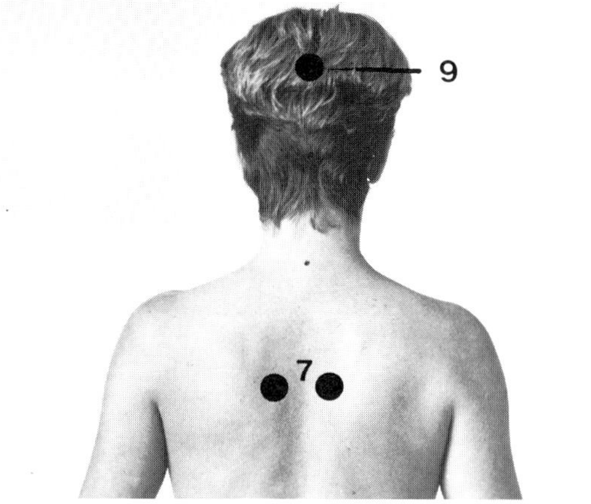


**Point 6**
(St. 36) Left and right
Positioned on the shinbone, 3 fingerbreadths below the knee. This point can also be found by laying the outstretched hand on the side of the knee. The point is at the place where the tip of the middle finger touches the leg.

**Point 7**
(B. 15) Left and right
Located in the 5th intercostal cavity, 2 fingerbreadths away from the midline of the body.

**Point 8**
(C.V. 15)
Located at the tip of the xiphoid process.

**Point 9**
(G.V. 19)
Located on the midline of the body at the back of the head, at the position where the occipital fontanel can be felt.

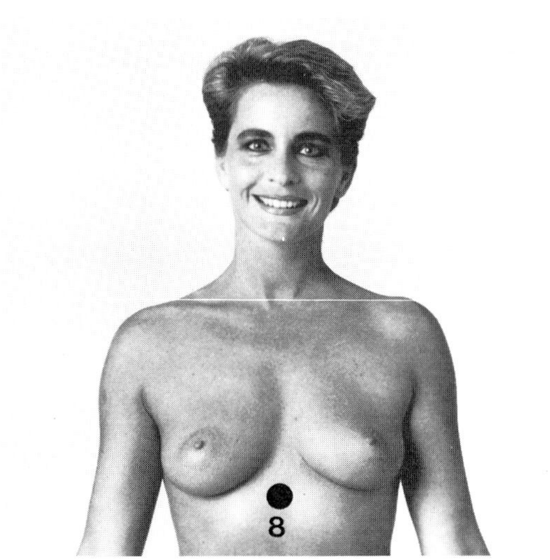

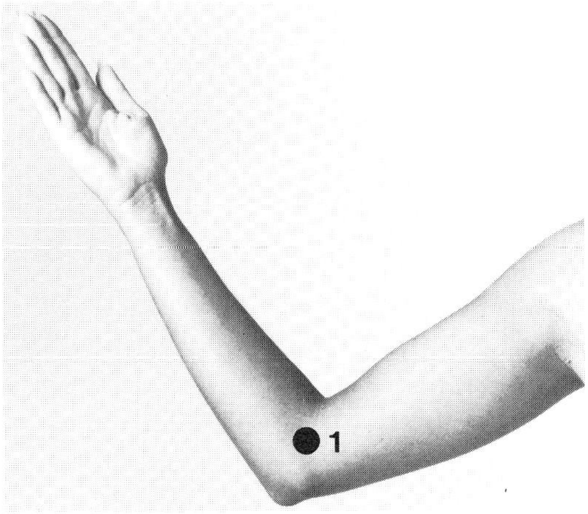


**Point 1** (H. 3) Left and right
Located at the medial end of the elbow crease.

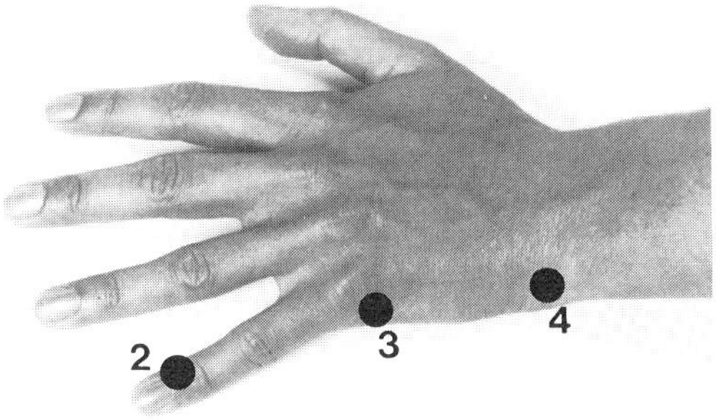


**Point 2** (H. 9) Left and right
Located on the medial side of the little finger, approx. 2 mm at a diagonal angle from the nailbed groove.

**Point 3** (S.I. 3) Left and right
Located above the basal joint of the little finger, at the end of the crease that occurs when the hand is slightly clenched.

**Point 4** (S.I. 4) Left and right
Located in the small gap between wrist and hand.

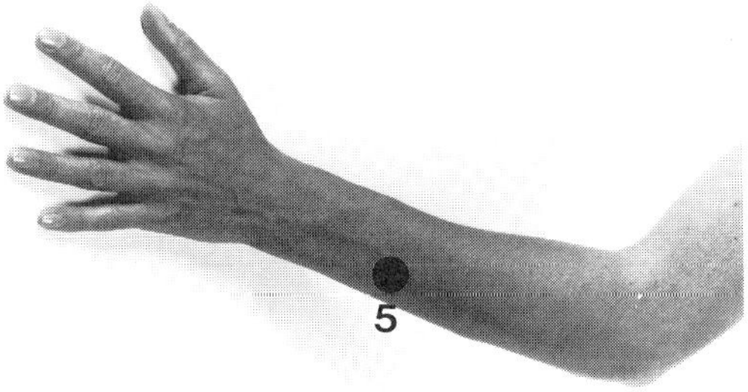


**Point 5**
(S.I. 7) Left and right
Located in the middle of the lateral side of the forearm.

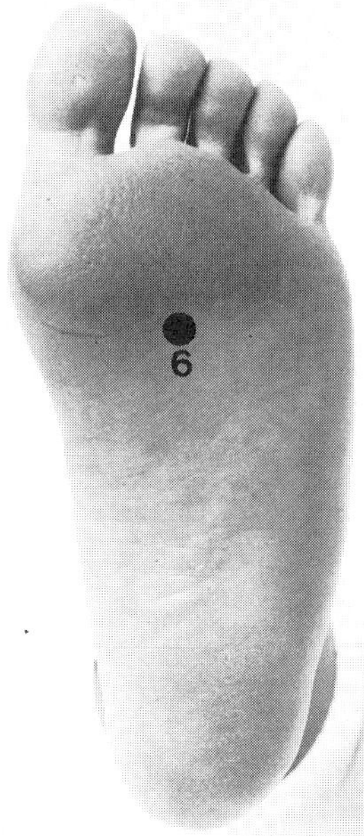


**Point 6**
(K. 1) Left and right
Located on the sole of the foot, between the ball of the large toe and the ball of the little toe.

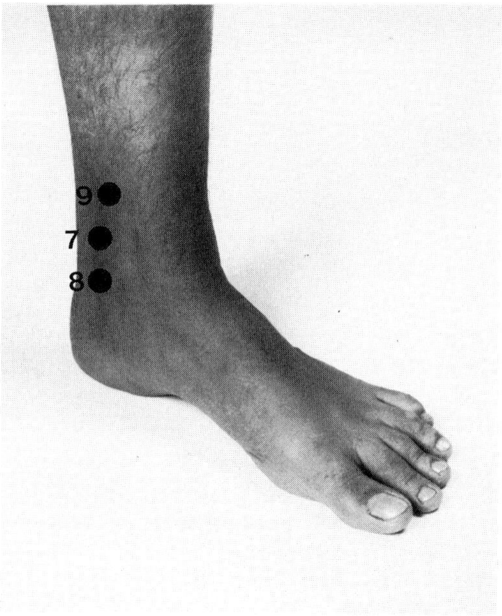


**Point 7**
(K. 3) Left and right
Located 1 fingerbreadth behind the medial ankle, between the Achilles tendon and the tip of the ankle.

**Point 8**
(K. 4) Left and right
Located approx. 2 fingerbreadths behind the medial ankle at a diagonal angle.

**Point 9**
(K. 8) Left and right
Located at the inner edge of the shinbone, approx. 2 fingerbreadths above the medial ankle.

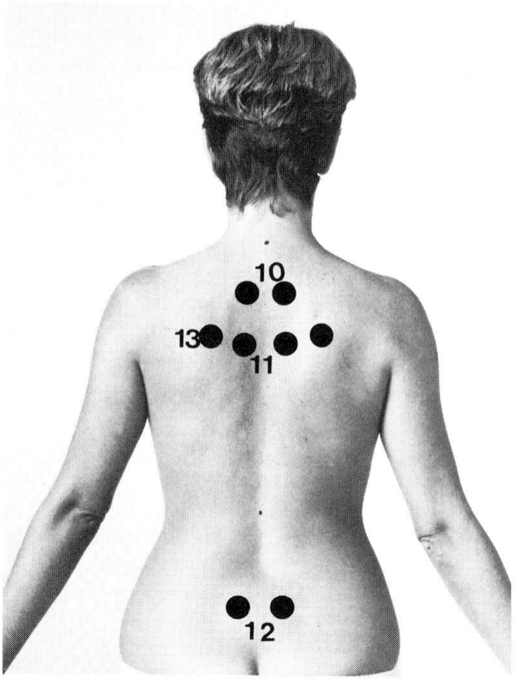


**Point 10**
(B. 13) Left and right
Located 2 fingerbreadths below the lateral ankle.

**Point 11**
(B. 15) Left and right
Located in the 5th intercostal space, 2 fingerbreadths away from the midline of the body.

**Point 12**
(B. 31) Left and right
Located on the medial side of the 1st sacral canal.

**Point 13**
(B. 39) Left and right
The left point is located in the 4th intercostal space, approx. 1 handbreadth to the left of the midline of the body, while the right point is located approx. 1 handbreadth to the right of the midline. The points are easy to find when the shoulders are pulled to the front.

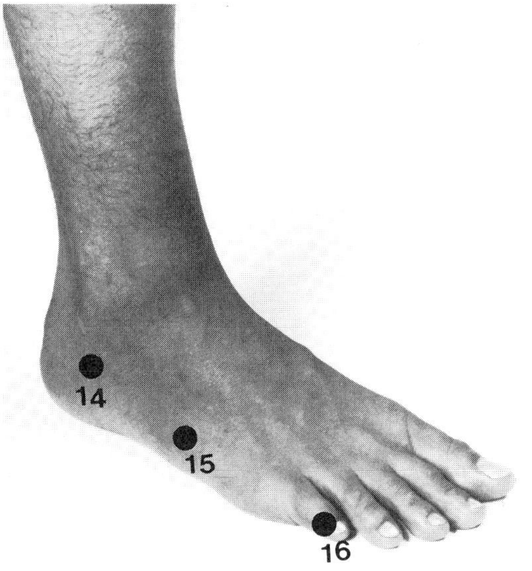


**Point 14**
(B. 62) Left and right
Located 2 fingerbreadths below the lateral ankle.

**Point 15**
(B. 64) Left and right
Located at the edge of the lateral side of the foot, at the end of the 5th metatarsal bone.

**Point 16**
(B. 67) Left and right
Located on the little toe, 2 mm away from the lateral angle of the nailbed groove.

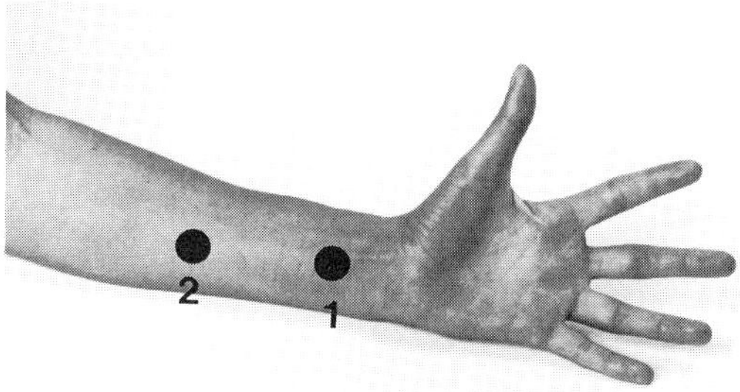


### Supplementary Points

**Point 1**
(C. 6) Left and right
Located in the middle of the medial side of the forearm, approx. 3 fingerbreadths above the first crease of the wrist.

**Point 2**
(C. 4) Left and right
Located exactly in the middle of the medial side of the forearm, slightly towards the bottom of the arm.

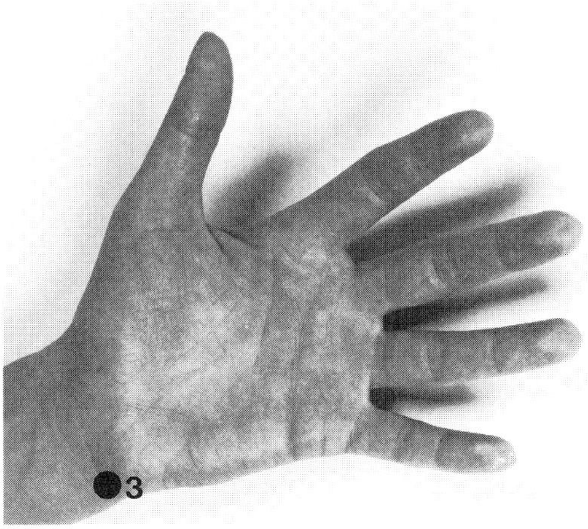


**Point 3**
(H. 7) Left and right
Located on the 1st crease of the wrist.

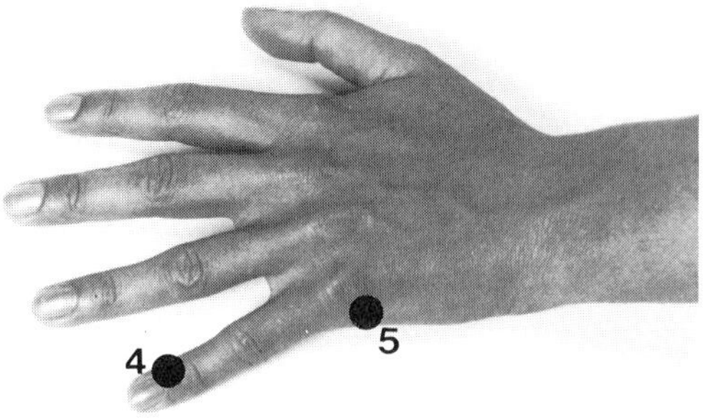


**Point 4**

(H. 9) Left and right

Located on the medial side of the little finger, approx. 2 mm at a diagonal angle from the nailbed groove.

**Point 5**

(S.I. 3) Left and right

Located above the basal joint of the little finger, at the end of the crease that occurs when the hand is slightly clenched.

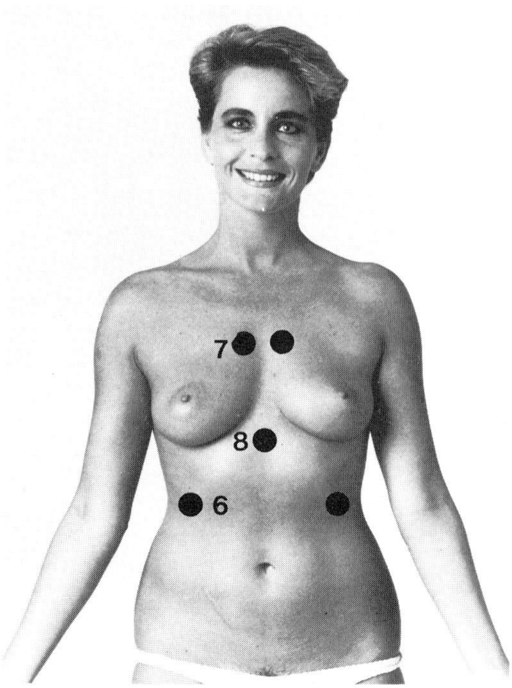


**Point 6**

(L. 13) Left and right

Located at a slight distance from the end of the lith rib.

**Point 7**

(K. 24) Left and right

Located next to the breastbone on the 3rd intercostal space, approx. 2 fingerbreadths away from the midline of the body.

**Point 8**

(C.V. 15)

Located at the tip of the occipital process.

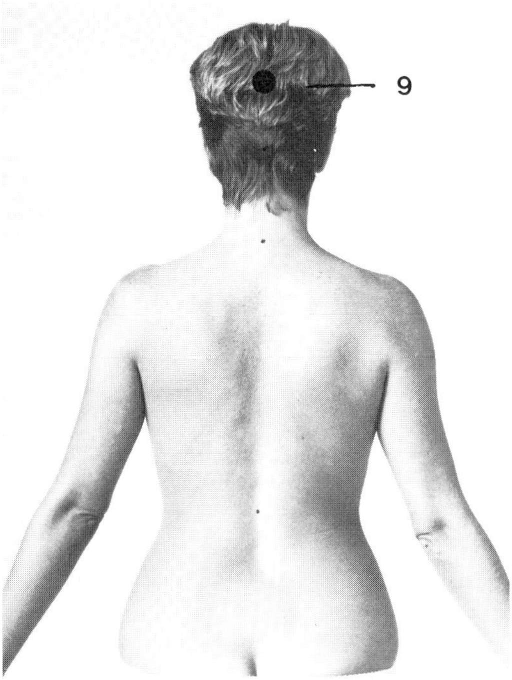


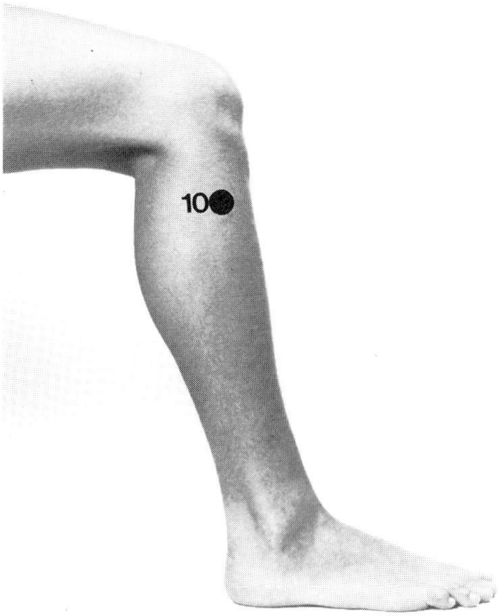


**Point 9**

(G.V. 19)

Located on the midline of the body at the back of the head, at the position where the occipital fontanel can be felt.

**Point 10**

(St. 36) Left and right

Positioned on the shinbone, 3 fingerbreadths below the knee. This point can also be found by laying the outstretched hand on the side of the knee. The point is at the place where the tip of the finger touches the knee.

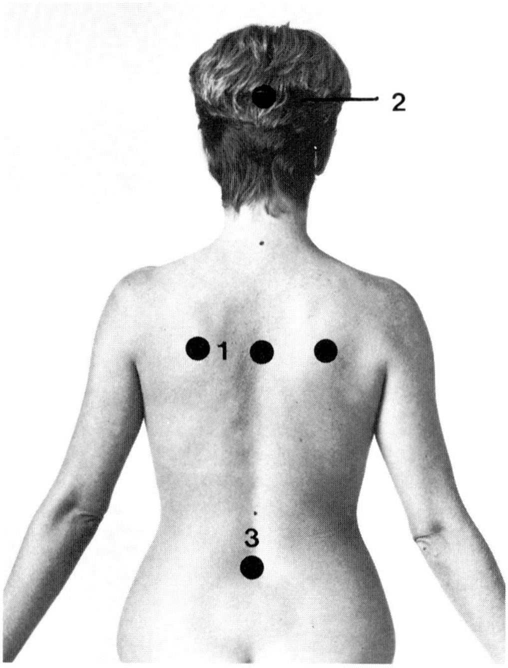


**Point 1**
(B. 39 – G.V. point – B. 39)
The first B. 39 point is located in the 4th intercostal space, approx. 1 handbreadth to the left of the midline of the body. The G.V. point is located on the spine itself and the left B. 39 point is located in the 4th intercostal space, 1 handbreadth to the left of the midline.

**Point 2** (G.V. 19)
Located on the midline of the body at the back of the head, at the position where the occipital fontanel can be felt.

**Point 3** (L5/S1)
Located on the midline of the body, between the spinal process of the 5th lumbar vertebra and the sacrum.

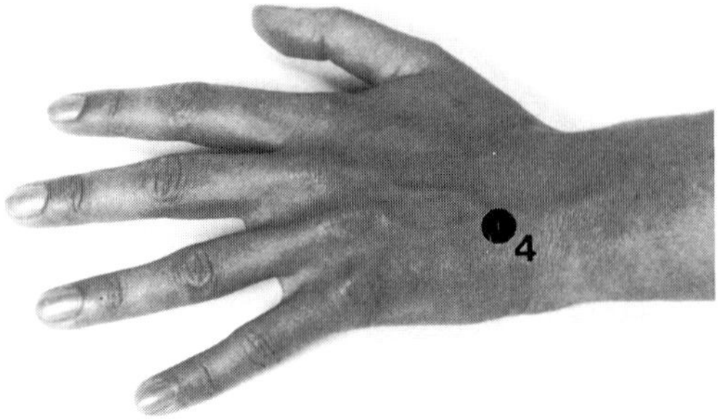


**Point 4**
(Psyche point of the left hand)
Lies at the point where the metacarpal bones end on the line leading from between the ring and the little finger.

During the course of my work with Kirlian photography, I have come across phenomena that indicate that there are also points in various zones and segments of the body. These include the so-called "regeneration" or "life" points, which have an extremely beneficial effect on physical and psychological well-being. Tiredness, weariness, exhaustion and even states of depression will react in a very satisfactory way to treatment with the acu-impulsor. All nine of the respective points should be marked on the body and treated with 10 impulses in consecutive order. Repeat three times, with a pause of two minutes between each treatment.

In order to locate the points, which are very easy to find since they are extremely sensitive, start out in the following way. First of all, look for the fourth point, which is located between the tip of the breastbone and the navel on the midline of the body. Points five and six are located approx. one fingerbreadth to the right and left of this point. Now draw an imaginary line around the body, on the level of point four. Point one is located on this point, in the middle of the spine. Points two and three are positioned one fingerbreadth above and below this point. Point seven is to be found in the middle of the cervical vertebra, with points eight and nine one fingerbreadth above and below it respectively.

These regeneration points can be treated in addition to all the other measures described in this book, and will also prove to be of benefit during times of health. They are especially effective when used in treatment of the previously described indications.

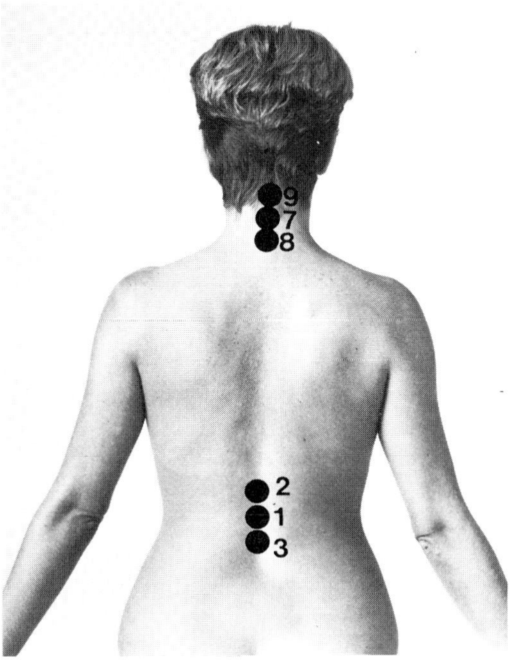


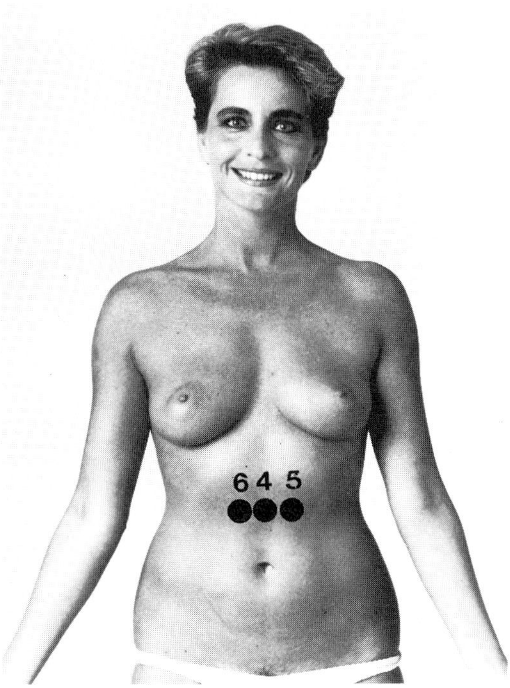

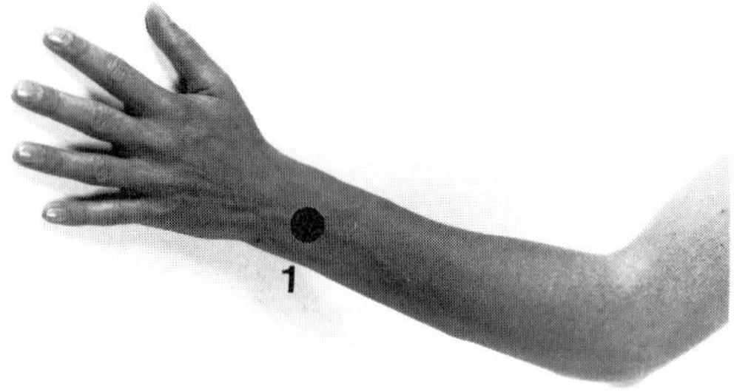


**Point 1**
(T.H. 3) Left and right
Located on the lateral side of the arm, between the ulna and the radius, approx. 2½ fingerbreadths above the fold of the wrist.

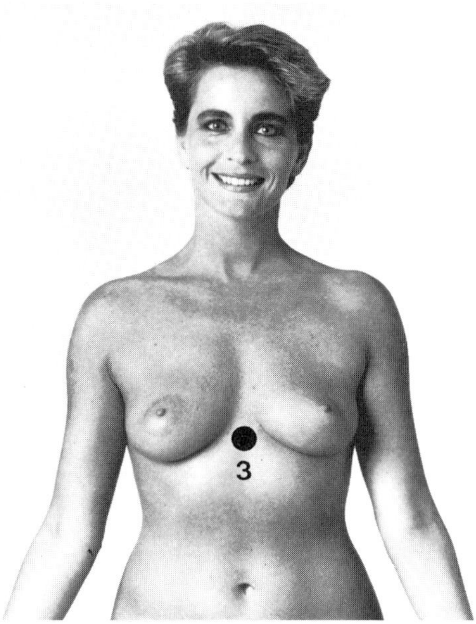


**Point 3**
(C.V. 15)
Located at the tip of the occipital process.

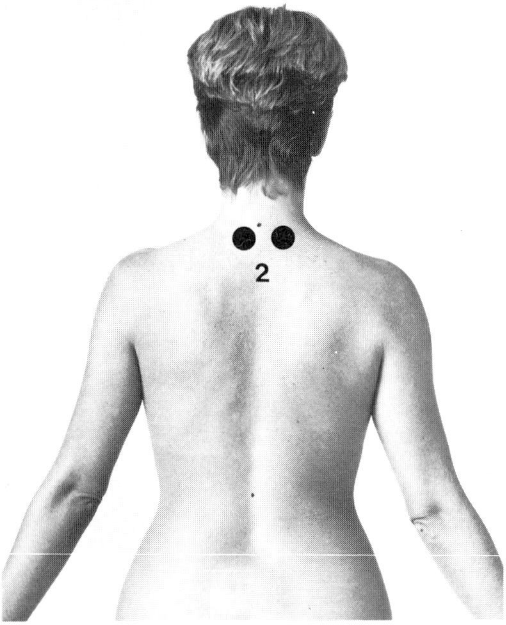


**Point 2**
(B. 11) Left and right
Located in the 1st intercostal space, 2 fingerbreadths away from the midline of the body.

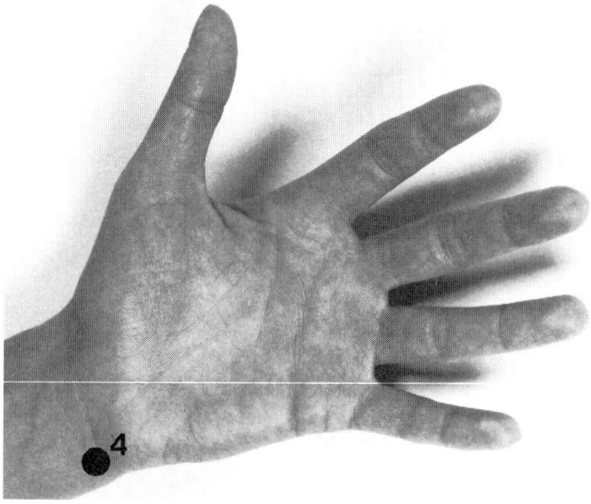


**Point 4**
(H. 7) Left and right
Located on the first crease of the wrist.

Despite the fact that medication is necessary in serious cases of arteriosclerosis, it is a measure which will only hold up the development of the disease but not bring about any fundamental changes. These have to be made in the areas that contributed towards the development of the disease in the first place, such as a wrong form of diet, lack of movement, excessive stress and the intake of nicotine.
In the treatment of arteriosclerosis, the use of the acu-impulsor as a supplementary measure will bring about excellent results. However, it must be kept in mind that treatment will have to be carried out daily over an extended period of time and that the factors mentioned above (false diet, lack of movement, etc.) will have to be changed. Treat each point with 10 impulses and repeat three times.

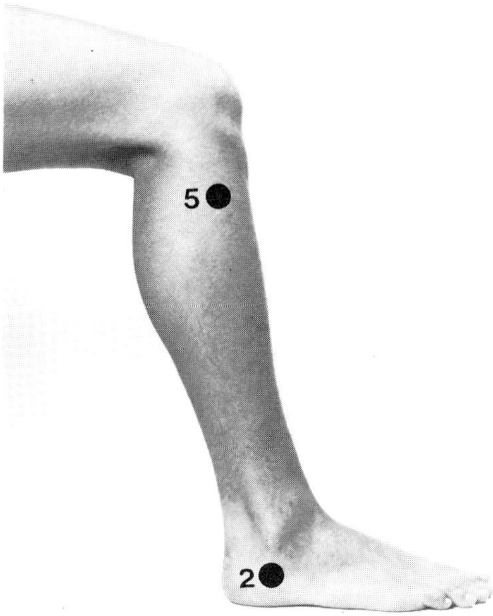


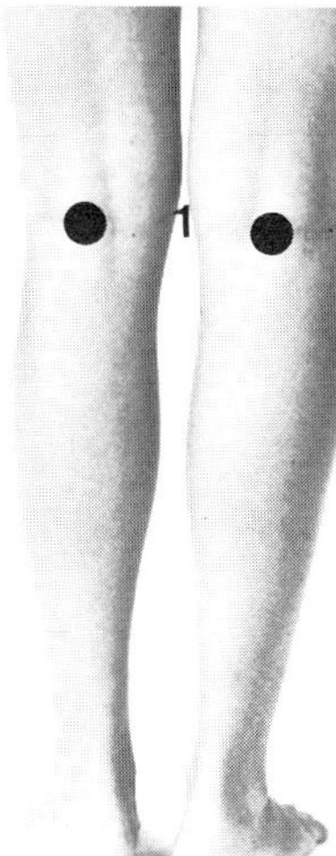


**Point 2**
(B. 62) Left and right
This point is located 2 fingerbreadths below the lateral ankle.

**Point 5**
(St. 36) Left and right
Positioned on the shinbone, 3 fingerbreadths below the knee. This point can also be found laying the outstretched hand over the side of the knee. The point is at the place where the tip of the middle finger touches the leg.

**Point 1**
(B. 54) Left and right
This point is located in the middle of the hollow of the knee.

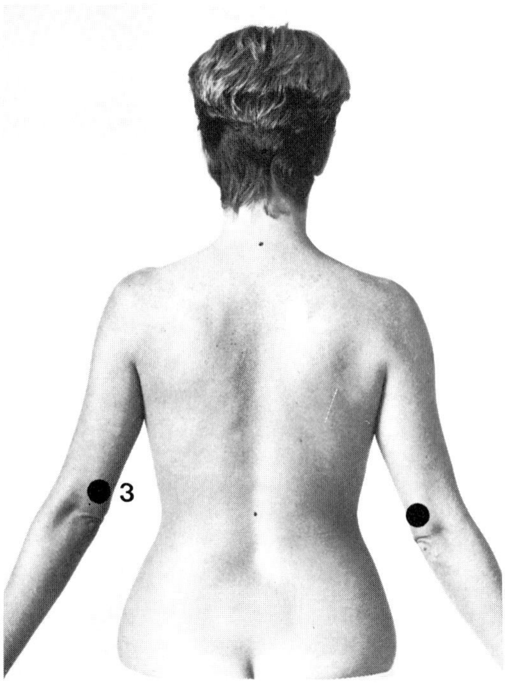


**Point 3**
(T.H. 10) Left and right
Located in the little hollow that can be found at the back of the arm when the elbow is bent.

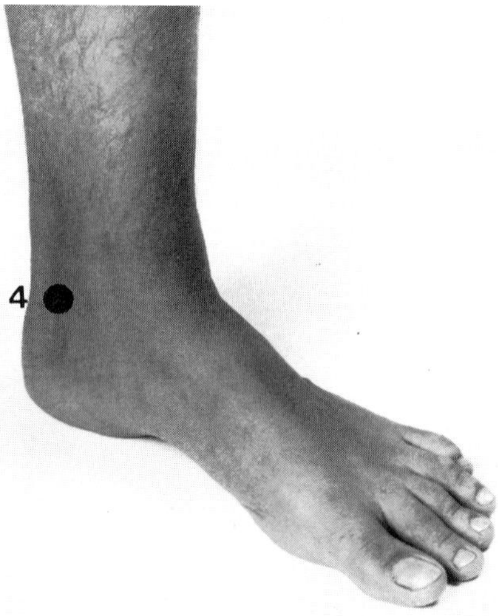


**Point 4**
(K. 3) Left and right
Located 1 fingerbreadth behind the medial ankle, between the Achilles tendon and the tip of the ankle.

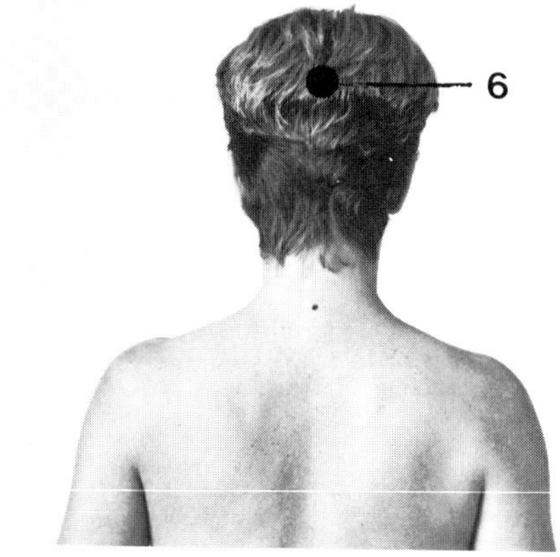


**Point 6**
(C.V. 19)
Located on the midline of the body at the back of the head, at the position where the occipital fontanel can be felt.

Dizziness can be caused by a number of diseases, ranging from simple circulatory disturbances and diseases of the inner ear to tumors of the brain. Therefore, as in the case of all illnesses, the cause must be diagnosed. If this does not prove to be of serious nature, you can take up treatment with the acu-impulsor (which is free of side-effects) while continuing with supplementary medication (which is not) for what will prove to be a short while. The basic therapy consists of eights points, which are treated daily. Once the condition begins to improve, treatment can be carried out less frequently until you end up with a rhythm of once every two weeks. If your dizziness occurs in combination with low blood pressure, treat the following points on one day and the points for dizziness with high blood pressure on the next in alternate fashion.

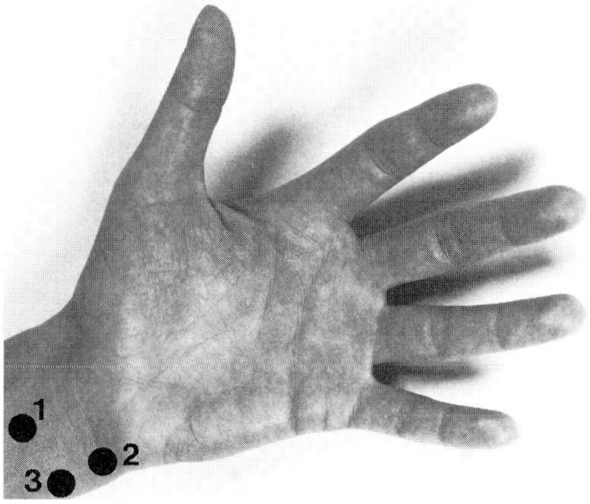


**Point 1**
(C. 6) Left and right
Located on the medial side of the forearm, approx. 3 fingerbreadths above the first crease of the wrist.

**Point 2**
(H. 7) Left and right
Located on the first crease of the wrist.

**Point 3**
(H. 5) Left and right
Located on the medial side of the forearm, 1 fingerbreadth above the crease formed by the wrist.

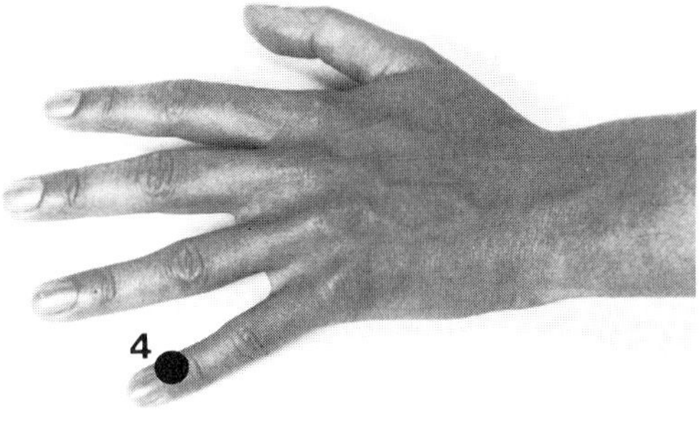


**Point 4**
(H. 99) Left and right
Located on the little finger, approx. 2 mm at a diagonal angle from the medial angle of the nailbed groove.

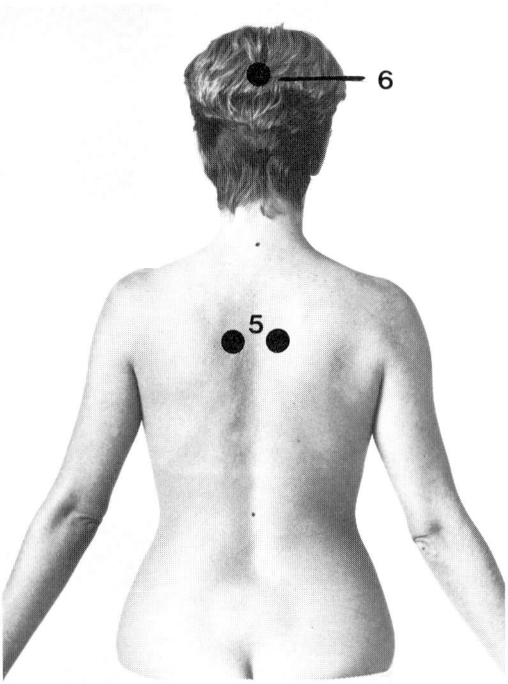


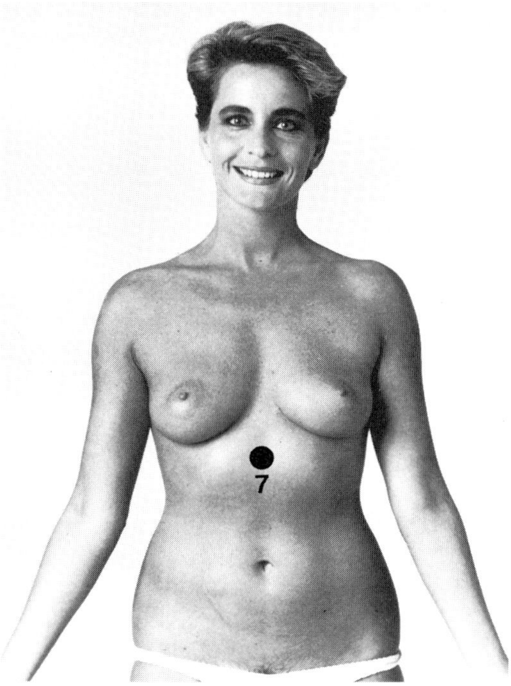


**Point 5**
(B. 15) Left and right
Located 2 fingerbreadths away from the midline of the body in the 5th intercostal space.

**Point 6**
(G.V. 19)
Located on the midline of the body at the back of the head, at the position where the occipital fontanel can be felt.

**Point 7**
(C.V. 14)
Located on the midline of the body, 1 fingerbreadth below the tip of the xiphoid process.

As a supplementary measure to medication, the following points can be treated in alternation with the previous ones for states of dizziness involving high blood pressure.

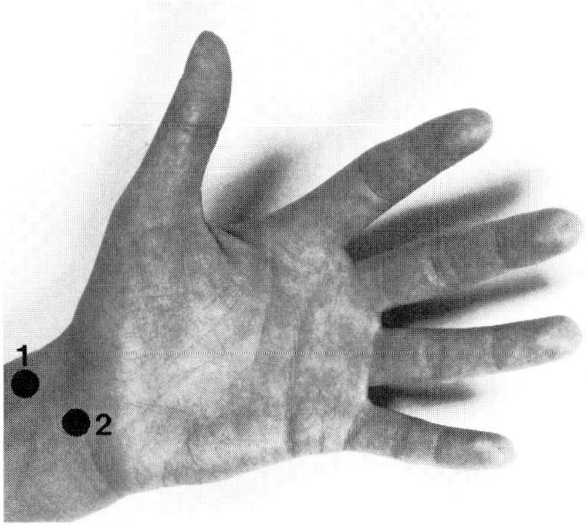


**Point 1**
(Lu. 7) Left and right
Located in the so-called radial groove, approx. 1 fingerbreadth away from the crease formed by the wrist.

**Point 2**
(C. 7) Left and right
Located on the medial side of the forearm, in the middle of the 1st crease formed by the wrist.

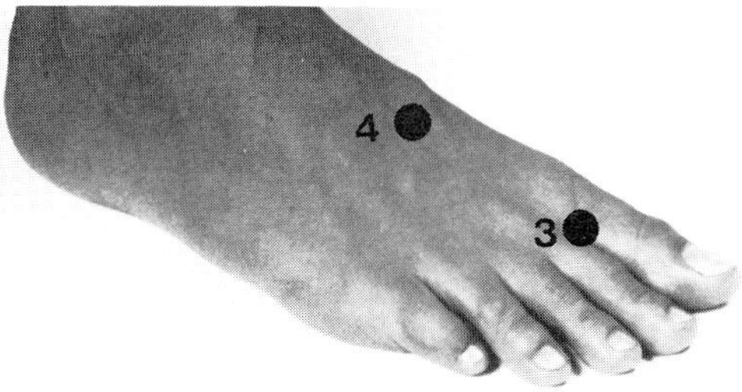


**Point 3**
(Liv. 2) Left and right
Located at the upper end of the skin formed by stretching the big and second toes.

**Point 4**
(Liv. 3) Left and right
Located on the lateral side of the end of the 1st metatarsal bone.

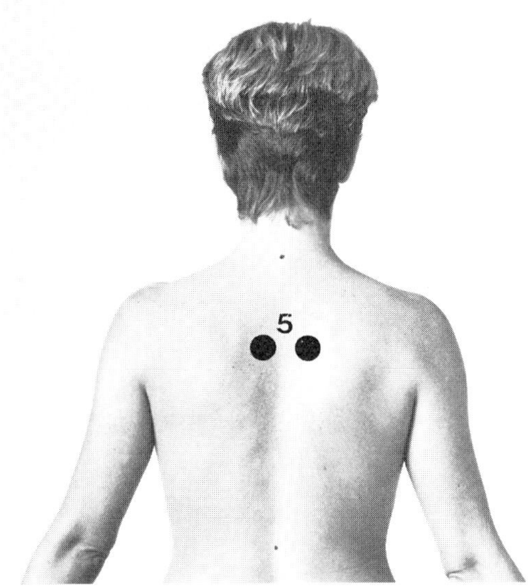


**Point 5**
(B. 14) Left and right
Located 2 fingerbreadths away from the midline of the body in the 4th intercostal space.

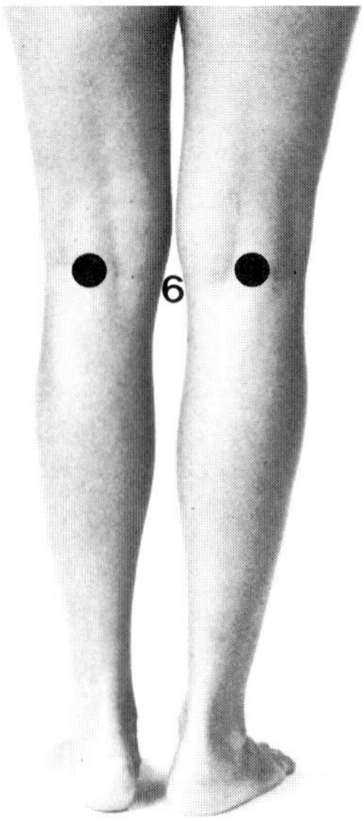


**Point 6**
(B. 54) Left and right
Located in the middle of the hollow of the knee.

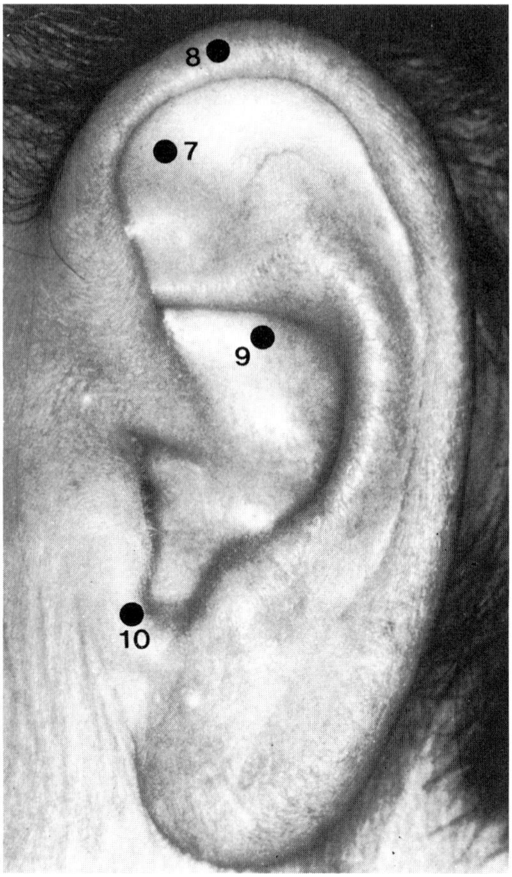


**Point 7** (Ear point 59)
**Point 8** (Ear point 78)
**Point 9** (Ear point 95)
**Point 10** (Ear point 19)

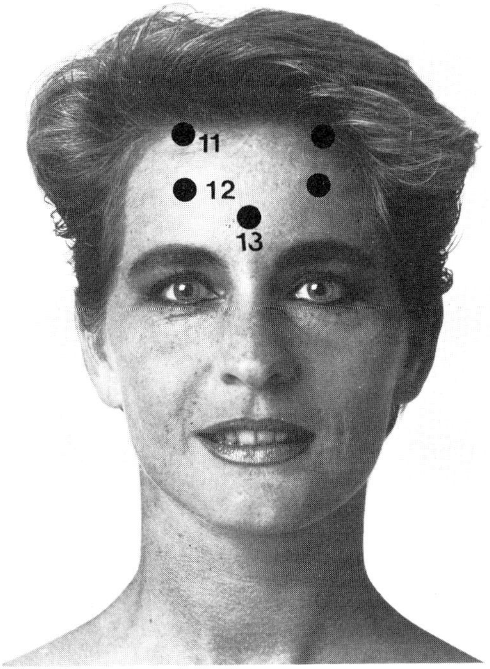


**Point 11** (Thalamus point)
**Point 12**
(Hypothalamus point)
Both points are located on a line leading up from the middle of the eye to the hairline. Palpate both points and treat the one that feels painful.
**Point 13**
(Limbic system)
Located 2 fingerbreadths above the point between the eyebrows. The second point is on the same line, 1 fingerbreadth away from the hairline.

When children wet their beds, the following thoughts should be taken into consideration:

1. Is the child suppressed in the family constellation; is it praised and cuddled sufficiently?
2. Has the child been examined to see whether there are organic causes for the condition, such as diseases of the urinary tract or abnormalities of the nervous system? Bedwetting can also be a symptom of juvenile-onset diabetes.
3. Is the diet correct?
4. Is the condition being caused by geopathological disturbances, such as water veins? In order to exclude this possibility, have the child's bed examined. Although many people regard this as mystical nonsense, tests carried out by cosmobiologists have proved that in addition to psychic factors, geopathological influences are one of the chief sources of bed-wetting in children.
5. Could undercooling be causing the condition? Is the child suffering from a cold in the bladder? In the case of babies and toddlers, these conditions can be caused by having to lie in wet diapers for too long.

In my opinion, most cases of bed-wetting are symptoms of a nervous or functional disturbance and can generally be healed with the help of the acu-impulsor.

I would like to stress the significance of water veins, for I have come across cases of bedwetting due to this cause again and again. It goes without saying that in such a case, the bed will have to moved to another place.

With regard to the treatment of cases of bedwetting, I would like to quote Dr. Mozer, who writes in his book *Brennpunkte der Krankheit*, published by Haug Verlag: "We have treated a considerable number of cases of bed-wetting with the focus method and were successful in every single case." The so-called focus massage consists of the vibrational massage of a point discovered by Dr. Mozer in the right groin. This point forms the basis of treatment of bed-wetting conditions with the acu-impulsor. Please proceed in the following manner.

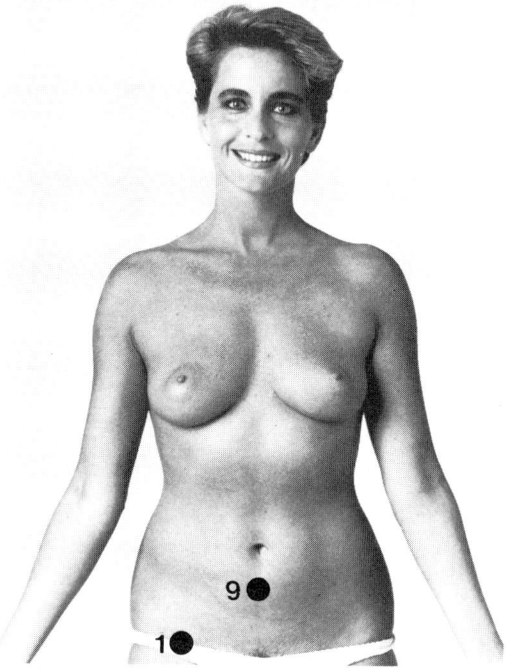


**Point 1**
Treat this point, which is located in the lateral third of the right inguinal region, with ten impulses. Repeat three times with a minute's pause between each treatment. Now treat points 9 and 10.

**Point 9**
(C.V. 6)
Located on the midline of the body, approx. 1 fingerbreadth below the navel.

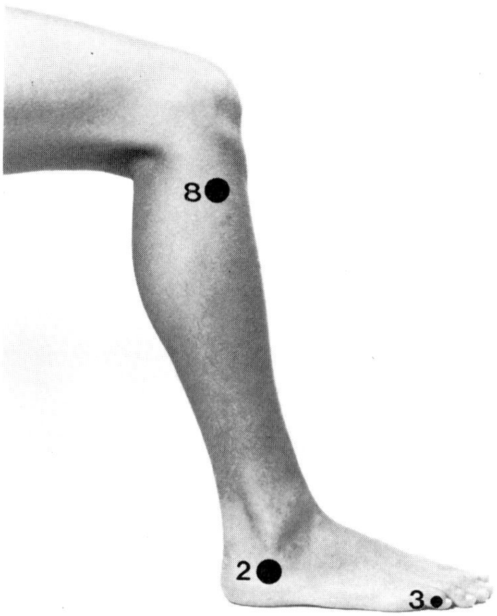


**Point 2**
(B. 62) Left and right
Located approx. 2 fingerbreadths below the lateral ankle.

**Point 3**
(B. 67) Left and right
Located at the lateral nailbed groove of the little toe, 2 mm away from the lateral angle of the nailbed groove.

**Point 8**
(St. 36) Left and right
Located on the shinbone, 3 fingerbreadths below the knee. This point can also be found by laying the outstretched hand on the side of the knee. The point can be found at the place where the tip of the middle finger touches the leg.

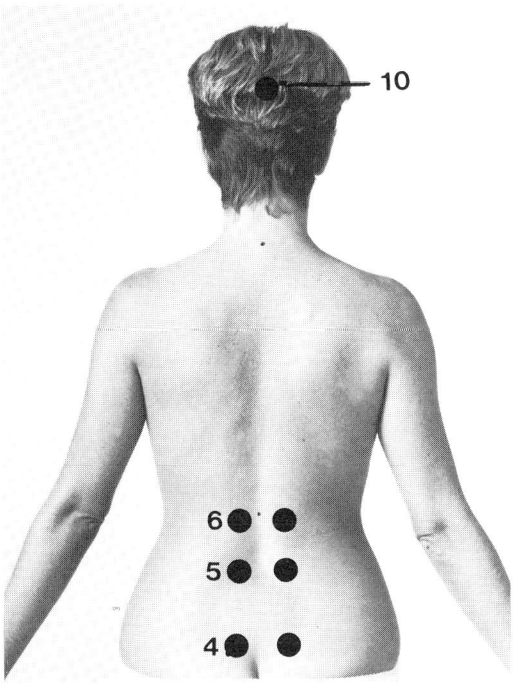


**Point 4**
(B. 28) Left and right
Located at the level of the sacral canal, approx. 3 fingerbreadths away from the midline of the body.

**Point 5**
(B. 25) Left and right
Located between the 4th and 5th lumbar vertebra, 2 fingerbreadths away from the midline of the body.

**Point 6**
(B. 23) Left and right
Located between the 2nd and 3rd lumbar vertebra, 2 fingerbreadths away from the midline of the body.

**Point 10**
(G.V. 19)
Located at the back of the head on the midline of the body, at the place where the occipital fontanel can be felt.

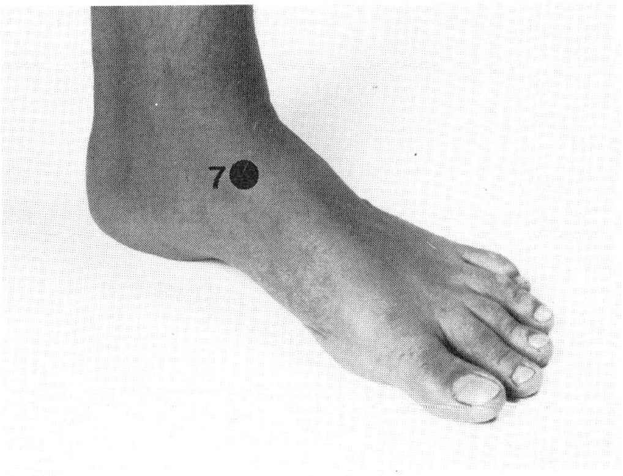


**Point 7**
(L. 4) Left and right
Located on the medial side of the tendon in the 1st ankle crease.

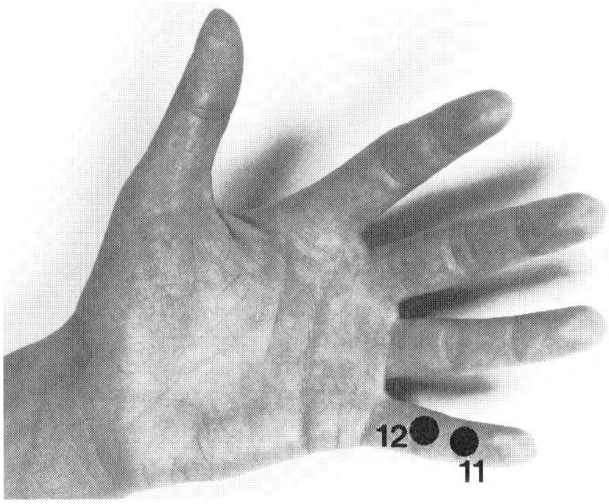


**Point 11**
(Hand point 1)
Located on the medial side of the little finger, in the middle of the crease closest to the fingertip.

**Point 12**
(Hand point 2)
Located on the medial side of the little finger, in the middle of the 2nd crease away from the tip of the finger.

In my work as a natural health practitioner, I am confronted daily with children who are physically and mentally underdeveloped. These nervous and pale-looking apparitions, almost transparent in effect, do not seem to be coming to terms with any aspect of their lives. Generally speaking, the psychic balance of these children has been disturbed by school pressure, troubles in the family and quarrels with siblings and friends. This results in poor school performance, a weak immune system, depression, lack of concentration, irritability and rejection by the parents.

When such children are brought to my practice, they can hardly articulate a single thought. Instead, they sit frightened and huddled up in their chairs, scared stiff of what is to come. I think it is extremely important to release these children from the clasps of negativity, and as has often proved to be the case, it isn't that difficult. Whether improvement is brought about with suitable homeopathic remedies, Colorpuncture or a combination of both is of no consequence as long as the method employed proves beneficial to the afflicted child.

In my opinion, however, home treatment with acu-impulse therapy will usually be entirely adequate, for the condition can generally be regulated to a satisfactory degree in this way.

This is because children are in a permanent state of development, which means that a small impetus is all that is generally needed to set the physical forces of self-regulation or self-healing into motion once again. In the case of these children, I feel that it is especially important to make sure that the difficult path that both they and all other children have to make though life in this day and age does not start off with illness. Indeed, the saying that the minor symptoms of youth develop into the serious complaints of adolescence and adulthood has lost none of its validity.

We should take it upon ourselves to explain the energetic and informational aspects of life to children. They generally understand it on an instinctual level and are able to cope with it in a manner that most adults would not believe possible.
However, it is not sufficient in the case of these children to simply have them treated by a doctor, or treat them at home with the acu-impulsor. This is because a number of other factors are just as important as the balancing-out of blocked energetic potential. But a start has to be made somewhere, and this can be done with acu-impulse therapy. In many cases, the children will soon be carrying it out themselves.

In the treatment of developmental disturbances, it will also be important to include the energy balancing programs 1 and 2 once or twice a week. I would like to point out once again that the organism of a child reacts far more swiftly to treatment than that of an adult. The following combination of points has proved to be very effective for children displaying symptoms of psychological disturbance, poor school performance and lack of concentration, general irritability and difficulties with parents and friends.

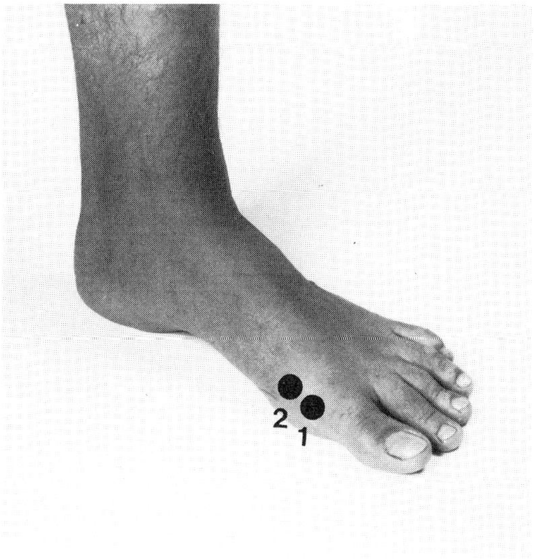


**Point 1**
(P. 2) Left and right
Located on the medial side of the basal joint of the big toe.

**Point 2**
(P. 3) Left and right
Located approx. 1 fingerbreadth away from the basal joint of the big toe.

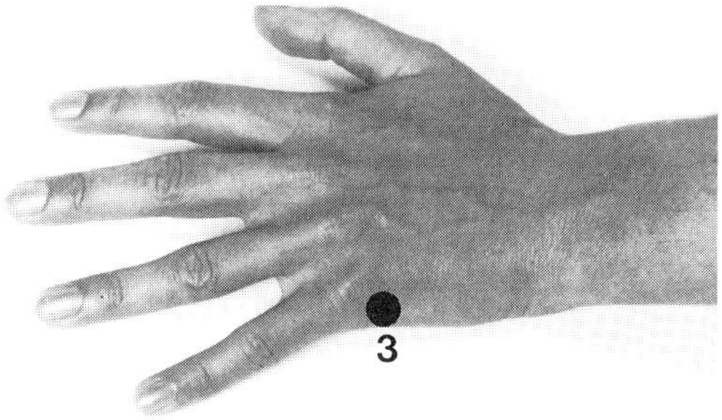


**Point 3**
(S.I. 3) Left and right
Located above the basal joint of the little finger, at the end of the crease that occurs when the hand is slightly clenched.

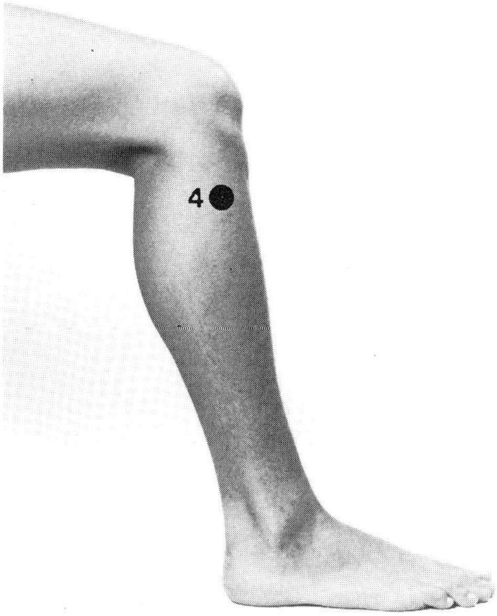


**Point 4**
(St. 36) Left and right
Located on the shinbone, 3 fingerbreadths below the knee. This point can also be found by laying the outstretched hand on the side of the knee. The point can be found at the place where the tip of the middle finger touches the leg.

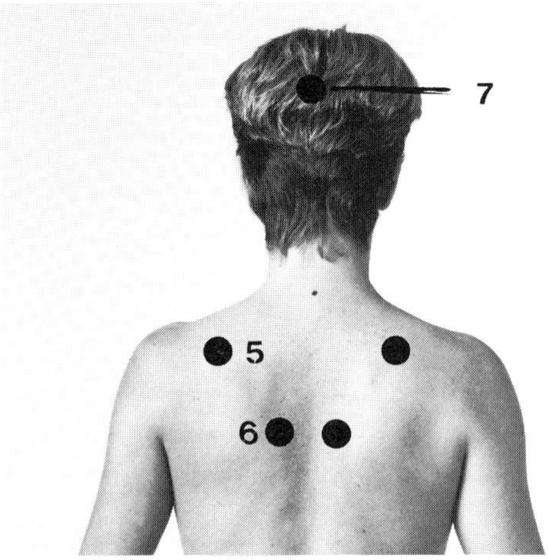


**Point 5**
(G.B. 21) Left and right
Located in the middle of the shoulder-blade, approx. 1 fingerbreadth away from the top edge of the same.

**Point 6**
(B. 15) Left and right
Located in the 5th intercostal space, 2 fingerbreadths away from the midline of the body.

**Point 7**
(G.V. 19)
Located on the midline of the body at the back of the head, at the position where the occipital fontanel can be felt.

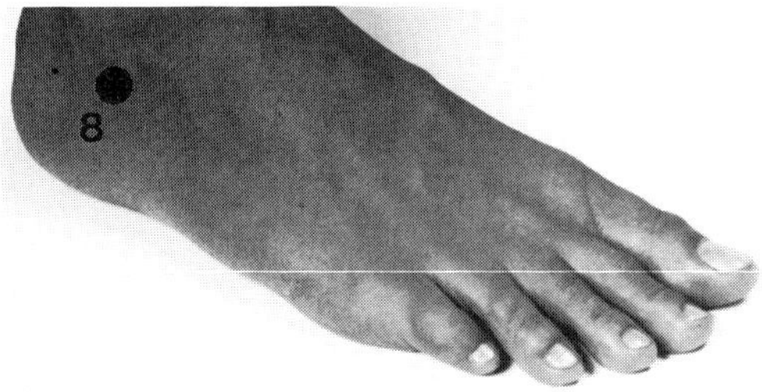


**Point 8**
(B. 62) Left and right
Located 2 fingerbreadths below the lateral ankle.

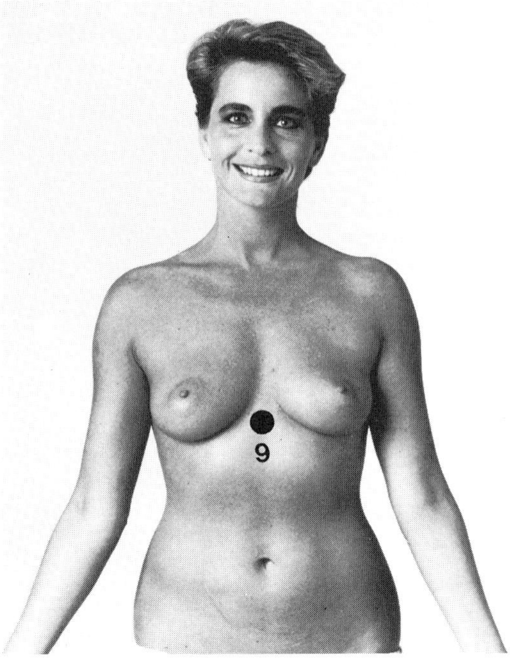


**Point 9** (C.V. 15)
Located at the tip of the xiphoid process.

These points should be treated twice a week, whereby the following routine has proved to be very valuable:

| | |
|---|---|
| Monday: | Energy balancing program 1 |
| Tuesday: | Treatment of the above-described points. |
| Wednesday: | No treatment |
| Thursday: | Energy balancing program 2 |
| Friday: | Treatment of the above-described points. |
| Saturday: | No treatment |
| Sunday: | No treatment |

Once you notice that the child is beginning to change in a positive way, the above-mentioned points need only need be treated once a week, along with both energy balancing programs. Later on, it will be sufficient to carry out this procedure once a month.

# Acute and Chronic Sinus Affections

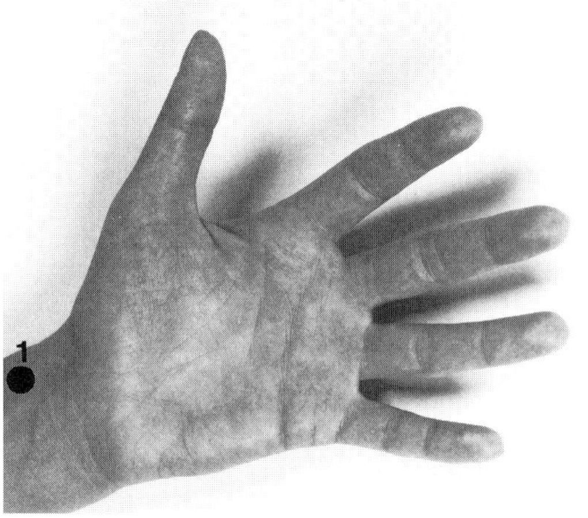


**Point 1**
(Lu. 7) Left and right
Located in the radial groove, approx. 2 fingerbreadths away from the fold of the wrist.

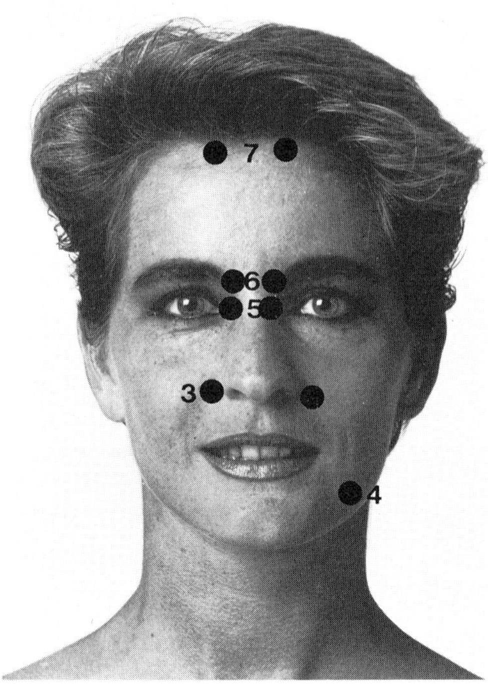


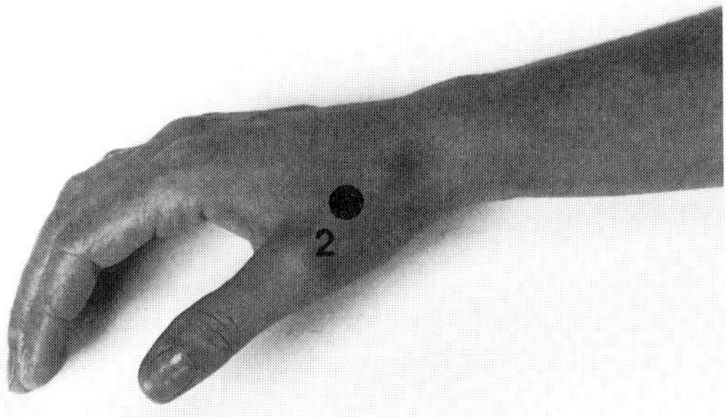


**Point 2**
(L.I. 4) Left and right
Located on the lateral surface of the index finger, where the metacarpal bones of thumb and index finger form an angle.

**Point 3**
(L.I. 20) Left and right
Situated on each side of the nostrils, directly on the nasolabial groove.

**Point 4**
(St. 5) Left and right
Located in the middle of the margin of the lower jaw above a small hollow.

**Point 5**
(U.B. 1) Left and right
Located at the internal corner of the eye.

**Point 6**
(U.B. 2) Left and right
Located at the medial end of the eyebrow.

**Point 7**
(U.B. 3) Left and right
Situated on the hairline, 2 fingerbreadths away from the midline of the body.

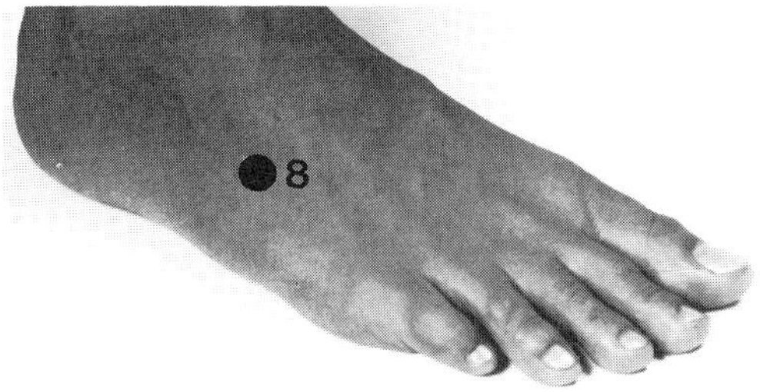


**Point 8**
(G.B. 41) Left and right
Located on the back of the foot on the distal end of the 4th and 5th metatarsals.

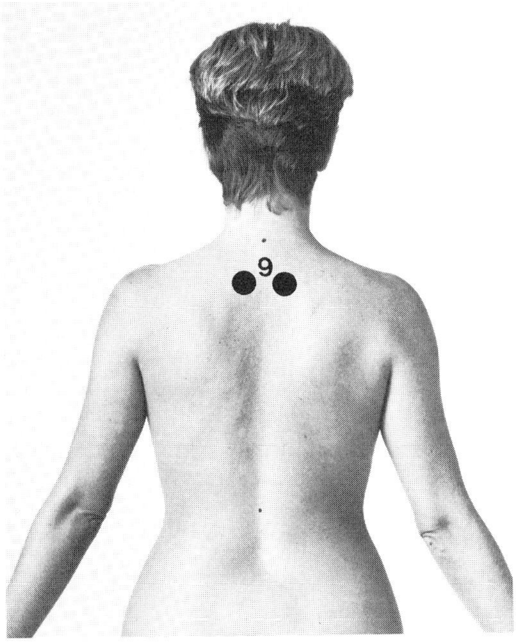


**Point 9**
(U.B. 12) Left and right
Located in the second intercostal space, 2 fingerbreadths away from the midline of the body.

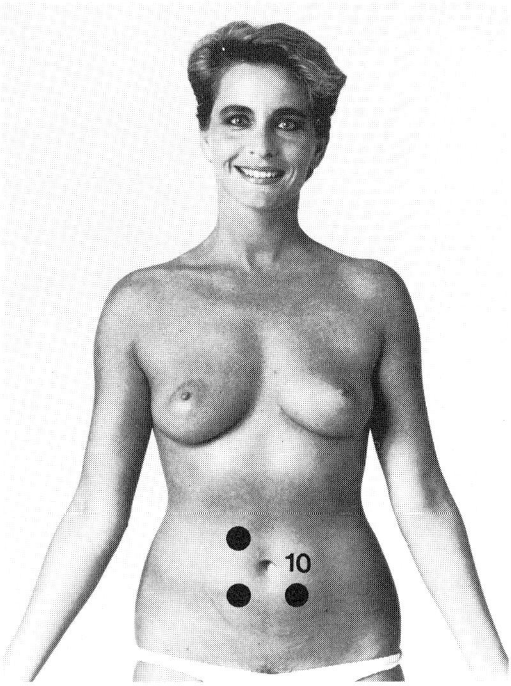


**Point 10**
(Aggressive zones)
Draw two diagonal lines intersecting the navel at a 45 degree angle. The first point is located to the left below the navel, 2 fingerbreadths away from the former. The second point lies in a similar manner to the right below the navel, while the third is located on the diagonal line to the left above the navel, two fingerbreadths away from the navel.

In all acute and chronic complaints of the sinuse it is essential for therapy to include other related areas of the body. Practitioners of natural therapeutics have always known that the intestinal tract plays an important part in many diseases. In many cases of sinus complaints the intestinal tract is a contributing factor. Therefore acu-impulsor therapy always includes the points which act on the intestinal tract.

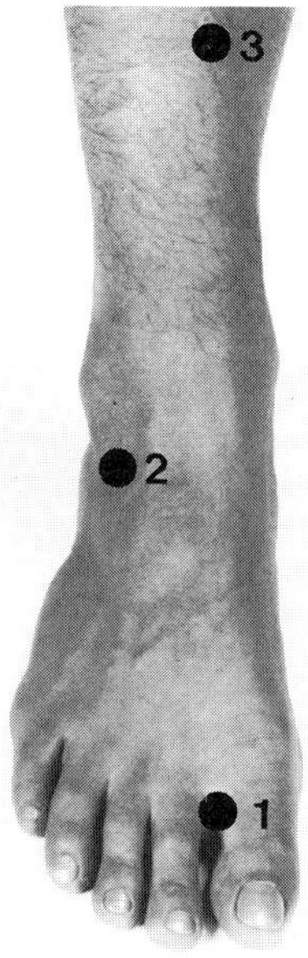


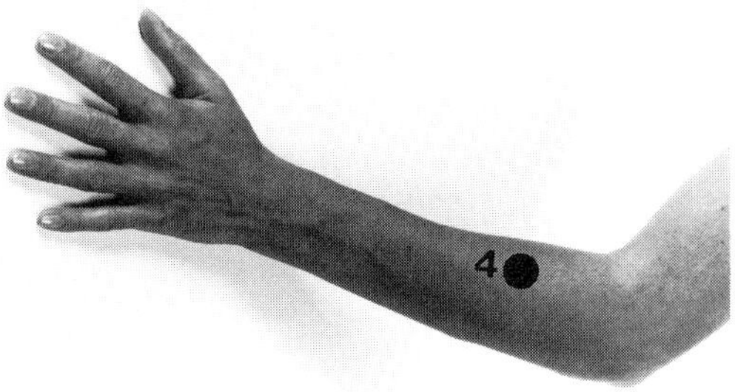


**Point 4**
(L.I. 10) Left and right
Situated on the medial surface of the forearm, 2 fingerbreadths below the elbow fold. This point will be found to be very painful and is therefore quite easy to locate.

**Point 1**
(Liv. 2) Left and right
Located on the upper margin of the web between the slightly spread 1st and 2nd toe.

**Point 2**
(G.B. 40) Left and right
Located on the back of the foot in a small hollow beneath the lateral malleolus.

**Point 3**
(Liv. 6) Left and right
Located at the midpoint of the shin bone on the medial margin.

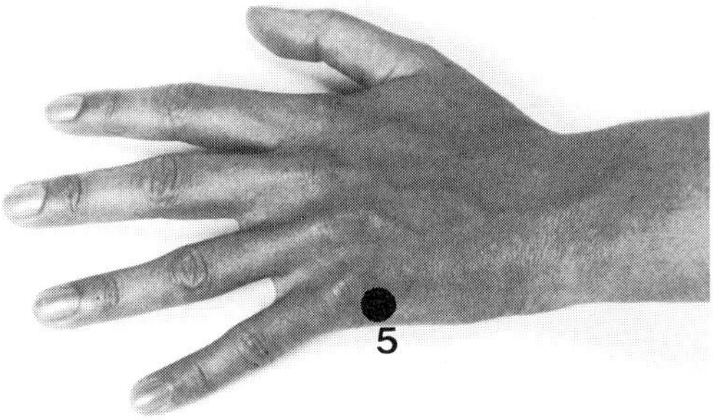


**Point 5**
(S.I. 3) Left and right
Located above the basal joint of the small finger at the end of a small fold which is formed by making a fist.

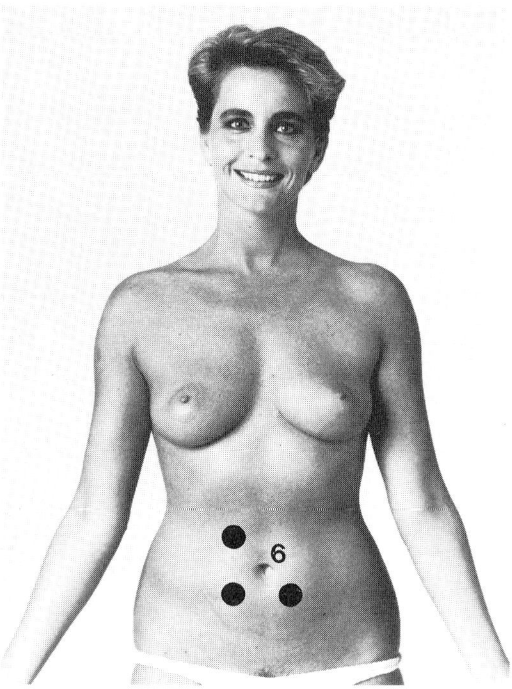


**Point 6**

(Aggressive zones)

Draw two diagonal lines intersecting the navel at a 45 degree angle. The first point is located to the left below the navel, 2 fingerbreadths away from the former. The second point lies in a similar manner to the right below the navel, while the third is located on the diagonal line to the left above the navel, two fingerbreadths away from the navel.

## Acute cases: evening

- Treat the points specified for acute and chronic sinusitis.

Once the complaints are improving, extend the intervals at which therapy is carried out until you are only treating the points once a week in the morning and evening.

## Chronic sinusitis

In chronic cases the previously specified points are treated twice a week. According to a therapeutic rule in natural healing, chronic symptoms must return to an acute stage before they can finally be cured. In the course of the treatment chronic symptoms can become acute again. In such a case carry out the treatment daily until improvement sets in. The treatment of chronic sinusitis requires the application of ten impulses per point according to the given order, twice weekly.

# Diseases of the Gastro-Intestinal Tract

1. Constipation
2. Ulcus Ventriculi (Gastric Ulcer)
3. Ulcus Duodeni (Duodenal Ulcer)
4. Heartburn
5. Diseases of the Gallbladder
6. Intestinal Cramps
7. Chronic Gastritis
8. Stomach Cramps

Diseases of the gastro-intestinal tract are extremely common in our day and age. They are often regarded as being minor complaints, although in most cases it can safely be assumed that they are part of a larger complex or syndrome of symptoms, as evidenced for example by individuals who are in a permanent state of nervousness or subject to severe stress and therefore experience gastro-intestinal symptoms such as pressure in the upper abdomen, sporadic bouts of diarrhea, constipation or sudden gastric pain. All these disorders will respond well to acu-impulsor treatment provided the causes are treated as well – i.e. point combinations for stress, anxiety and restlessness, etc. are included. Even in cases of more serious gastro-intestinal disorders acu-impulsor therapy often shows good results. Nevertheless the following combinations are intended as concomitant therapy. Regular application leads to rapid improvement in most cases. In all cases of gastro-intestinal diseases the other organs involved in the metabolic process must also be examined. In many instances complaints manifesting in the stomach or intestines may be caused by disorder of the liver, gallbladder or pancreas. Thorough diagnosis will bring such matters to light so that they can be treated accordingly.

The following combination is suited for bringing quick relief, particularly in the case of pain.

1. Energy balancing – Control 1, followed by the indicated point combination, Stomach – Intestines – Liver – Gallbladder.

I would like to point out that constipation is a serious disorder of which the effects are generally greatly underestimated. When one considers how many metabolic disorders are caused by the toxic states arising from chronic constipation, the significance of regular bowel movements will be obvious.

The long term use of laxatives is not without adverse effects of its own, therefore self-treatment with the acu-impulsor is an excellent way to cut down on medication and improve your health at the same time.

The following points are very effective and should be treated daily. As soon as the bowel movements begin to become more regular, the intervals between individual treatment should be extended until normal bowel movements occur without any therapeutic measures. It goes without saying that establishing a healthy, balanced diet with sufficient fiber, is a factor of considerable importance.

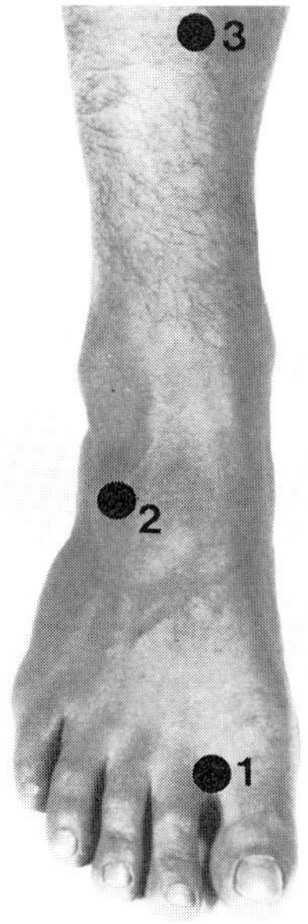


**Point 1**
(Liv. 2) Left and right
Located on the upper margin of the web between the 1st and 2nd toe when they are slightly extended.

**Point 2**
(G.B. 40) Left and right
Located on the back of the foot in a small hollow somewhat below and offset from the lateral malleolus.

**Point 3**
(Liv. 6) Left and right
Located at the middle of the shin bone, on the medial margin.

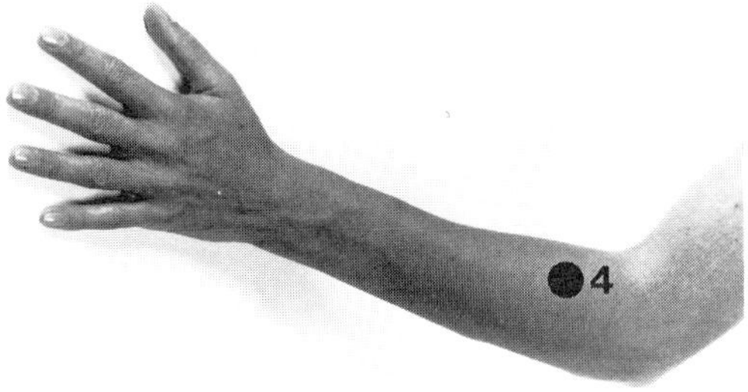


**Point 4**
(L.I. 10)
Situated on the medial surface of the forearm, 2 fingerbreadths below the elbow fold. This point will be found to be very painful and is therefore quite easy to locate.

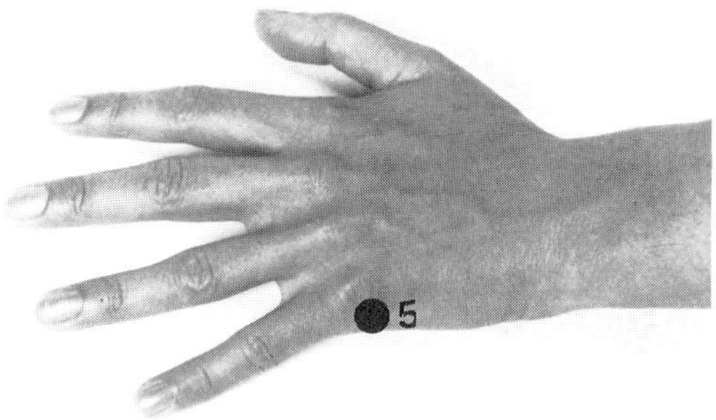


**Point 5**
(S.I. 3) Left and right
This point is located above the basal joint of the small finger at the end of a fold which appears when a fist is formed.

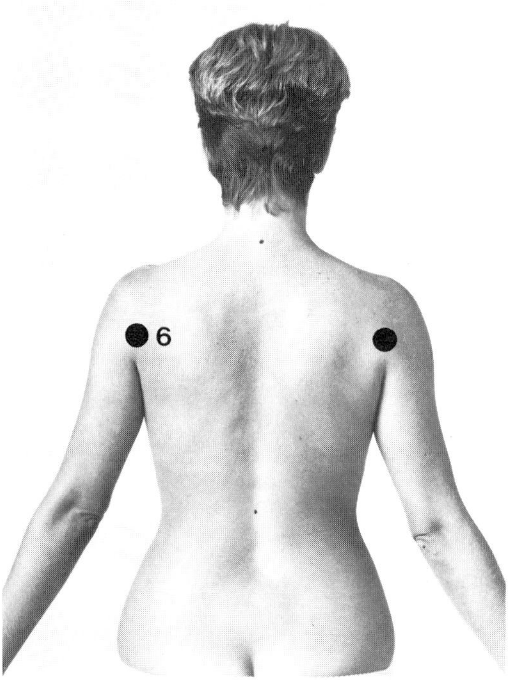


**Point 6**
(S.I. 9) Left and right
Situated 2 fingerbreadths above the axillar fold.

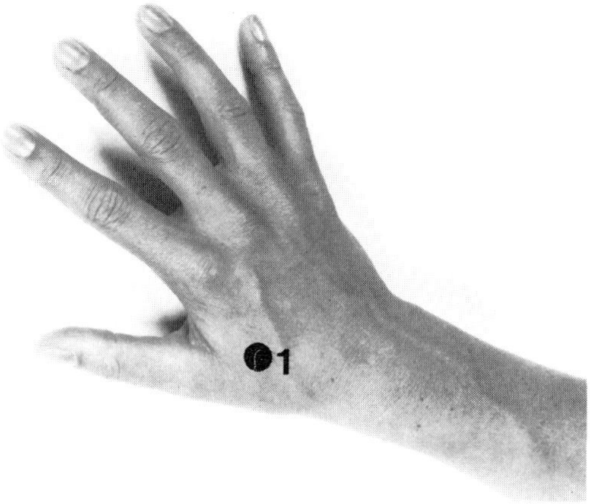


**Point 1**
(L.I. 4)
Located on the medial surface of the index finger in the angle where thumb and index finger converge.

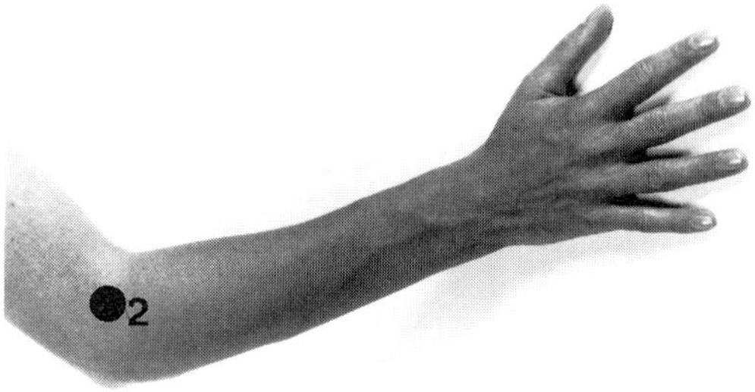


**Point 2**
(L.I. 11) Left and right
Located at the end of the external elbow fold.

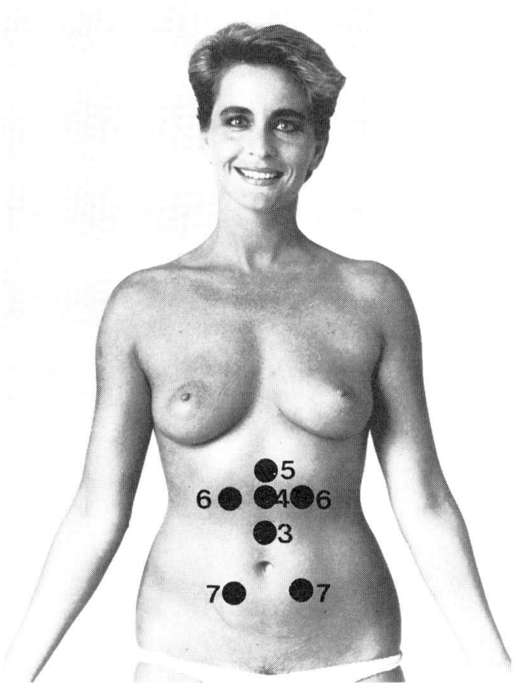


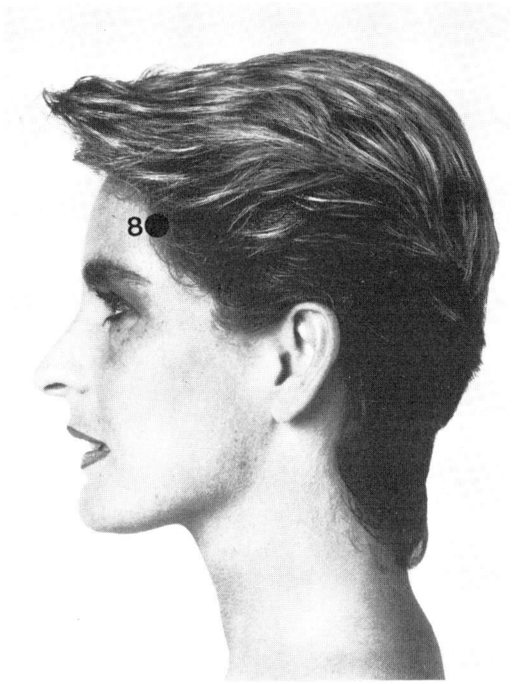


**Point 3** (C.V. 10)
Situated 2 fingerbreadths above the navel on the midline of the body.

**Point 4** (C.V. 12)
Located on the midline of the body exactly halfway between the navel and the tip of the xiphoid.

**Point 5** (C.V. 13)
Located 1 fingerbreadth above C.V. 12, on the midline of the body between the navel and the tip of the xiphoid.

**Point 6** (St. 21)
Located on the same level as C.V. 12, two fingerbreadths to each side of the midline of the body.

**Point 7 –** (St. 26) Left and right
Located 1 fingerbreadth below the navel and 2 fingerbreadths to each side of the midline of the body.

**Point 8**
(St. 1) Left and right
Located on the upper temple region, 4 fingerbreadths above and 1 fingerbreadth behind the orbital margin.

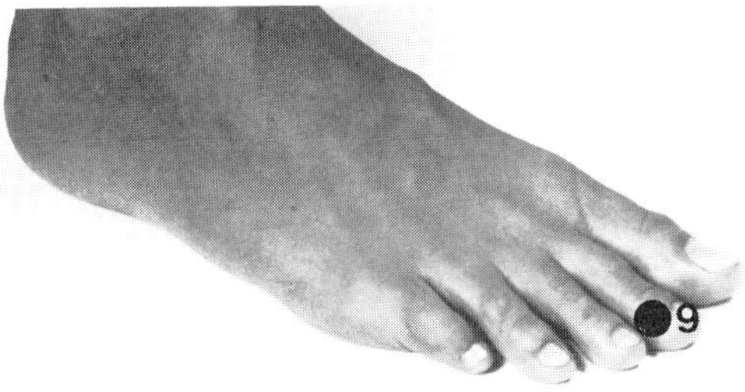


**Point 9**
(St. 45) Left and right
Situated on the lateral surface of the second toe, approx. 2 mm diagonally offset from the angle of the nailbed groove.

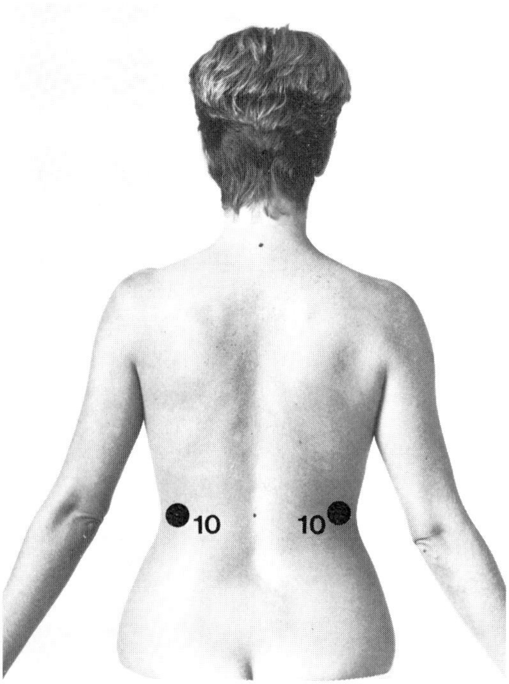


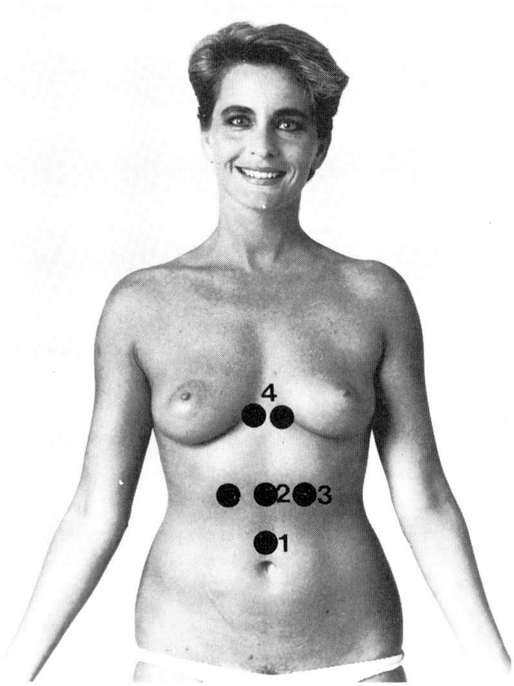


**Point 10**
(Posterior rib angle point – Pain point)
Located left and right on the lateral surface of the back, where a small hollow can be felt in the region of the ribs.

**Point 1**
(C.V. 10)
Situated 2 fingerbreadths above the navel on the midline of the body.

**Point 2**
(C.V. 12)
Located exactly in the middle between the navel and the tip of the xiphoid on the midline of the body.

**Point 3**
(St. 21) Left and right
Located approx. 2 fingerbreadths to each side of C.V. 12.

**Point 4**
(K. 21) Left and right
Located to both sides of the tip of the xiphoid, on level with the 6th intercostal space, ½ fingerbreadth away from the midline of the body.

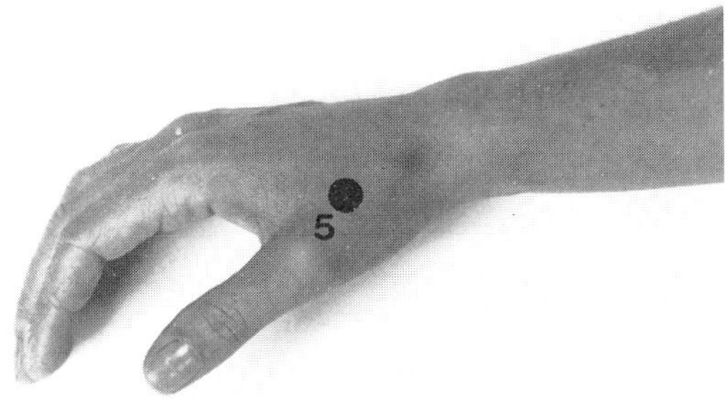


**Point 5**
(S.I. 4) Left and right
Located on the lateral surface of the index finger in the angle formed by the convergence of thumb and index finger.

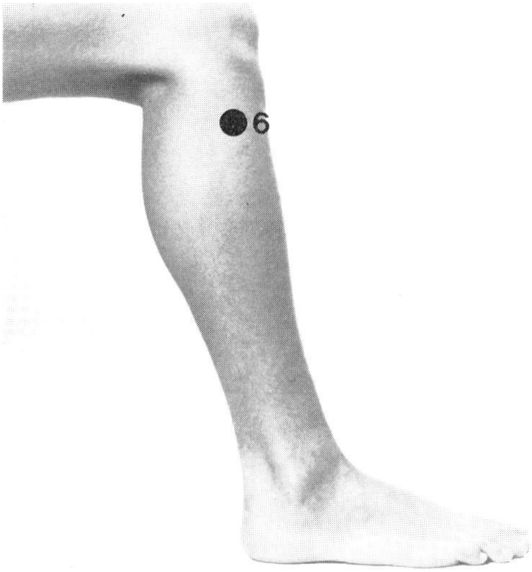


**Point 6**
(St. 36) Left and right
Located on the lateral, anterior surface of the lower leg, on the middle of the shin bone three fingerbreadths below the knee. This point can also be determined by placing the palm of the hand on the knee – the tip of the middle finger aims at the point.

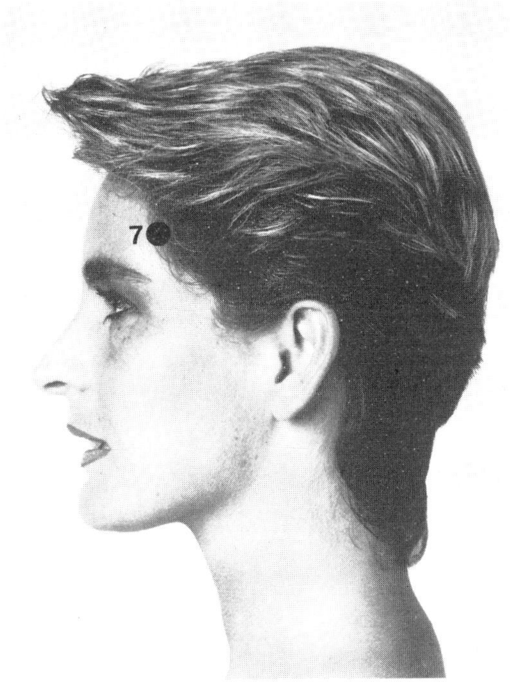


**Point 7**
(St. 1) Left and right
Located on the upper temple region, 4 fingerbreadths above and 1 fingerbreadth behind the orbital margin.

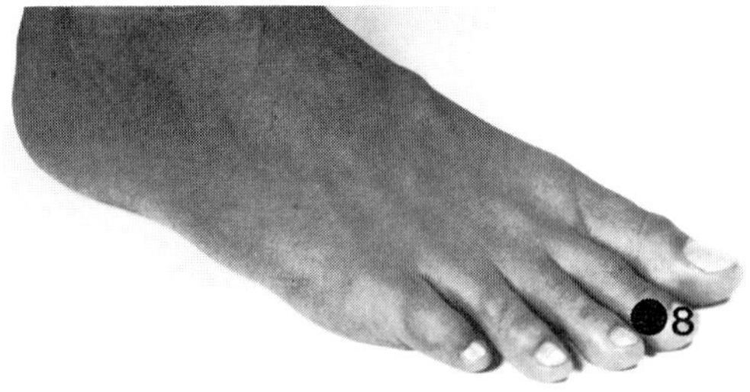


**Point 8**
(St. 45) Left and right
Located at the lateral nailbed groove angle of the 2nd toe, approx. 2 mm diagonally offset from the angle of the nailbed groove.

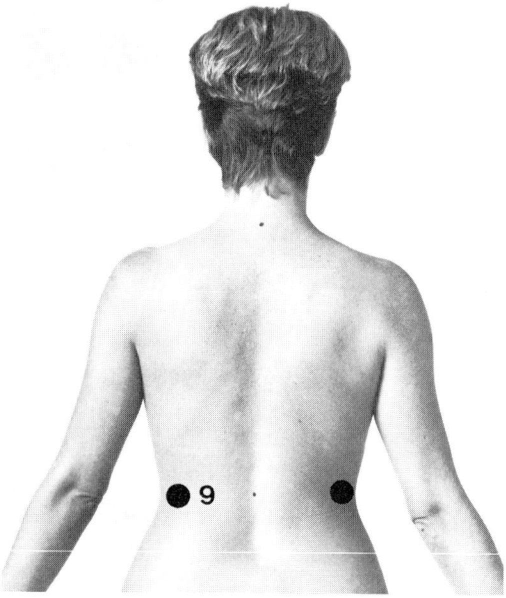


**Point 9**
(Rib angle point)
Located left and right on the lateral surface of the back where a small hollow can be felt in the region of the ribs.

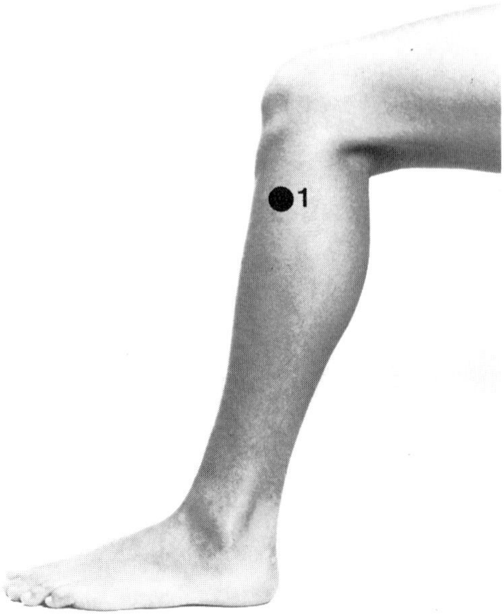


**Point 1**
(St. 36) Left and right
Located on the lateral, anterior surface of the lower leg, on the middle of the shin bone three fingerbreadths below the knee. This point can also be determined by placing the palm of the hand on the knee – the tip of the middle finger aims at the point.

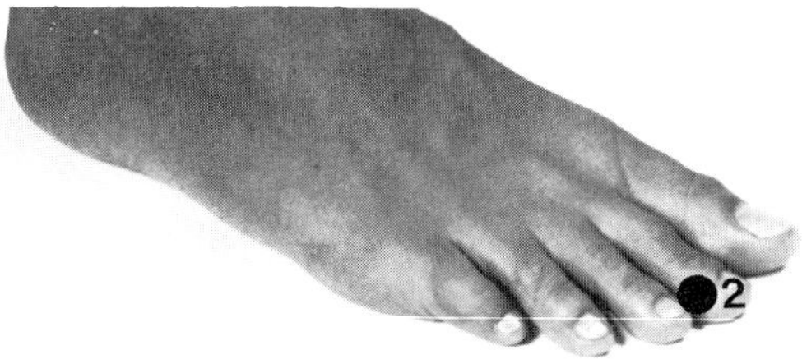


**Point 2**
(St. 45) Left and right
Located at the lateral nailbed groove angle of the 2nd toe, approx. 2 mm diagonally offset from the angle of the nailbed groove.

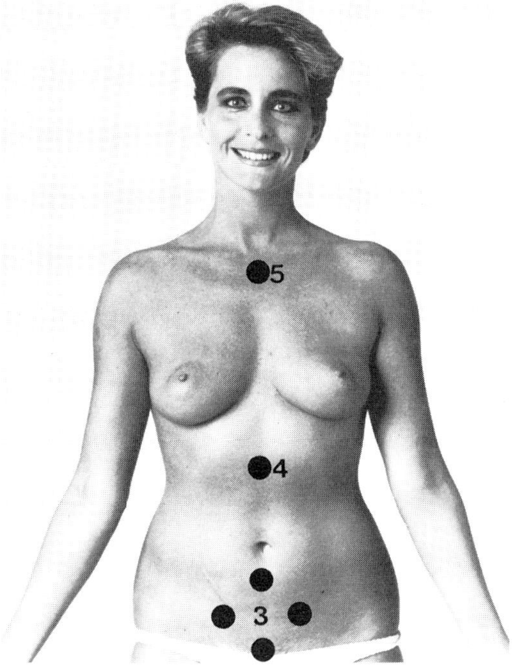


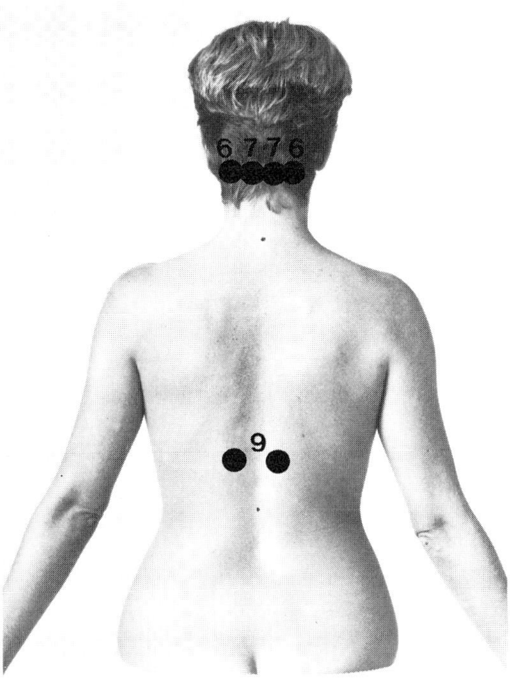


**Point 3**
(Abdominal rhombus)
The point on the pubic hairline and the one 2 fingerbreadths below the navel on the midline of the body form the vertical line, the points to the left and the right are situated 2 fingerbreadths from the midline of the body.

**Point 4**
(C.V. 13)
Located 1 fingerbreadth above C.V. 12 on the midline of the body.

**Point 5**
(C.V. 21)
Located on level with the 1st intercostal space on the midline of the body.

**Point 6**
(G.B. 20) Left and right
Located in a hollow 1 fingerbreadths below the lateral occipital protuberance and approx. 3 fingerbreadths away from the midline of the body.

**Point 7**
(U.B. 10) Left and right
Located approx. 1 fingerbreadth below the squamous part of the occipital bone and 1½ fingerbreadth away from the midline of the body. This point will be found to be painful to touch.

**Point 9**
(U.B. 21) Left and right
Located in the 12th intercostal space, 2 fingerbreadths away from the midline of the body.

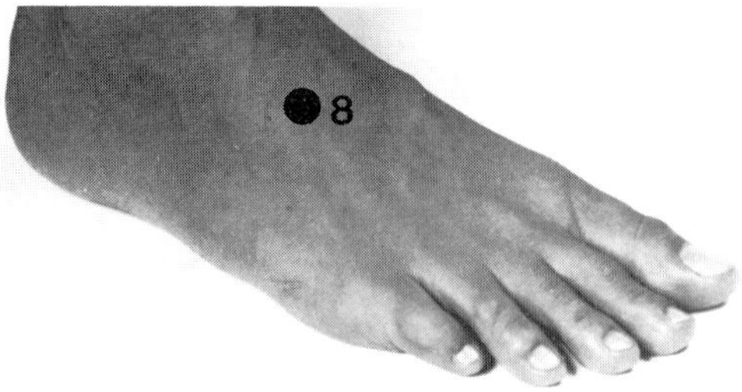


**Point 8**
(St. 42) Left and right
Situated on the back of the foot above the proximal end of the 2nd and 3rd metatarsal bones.

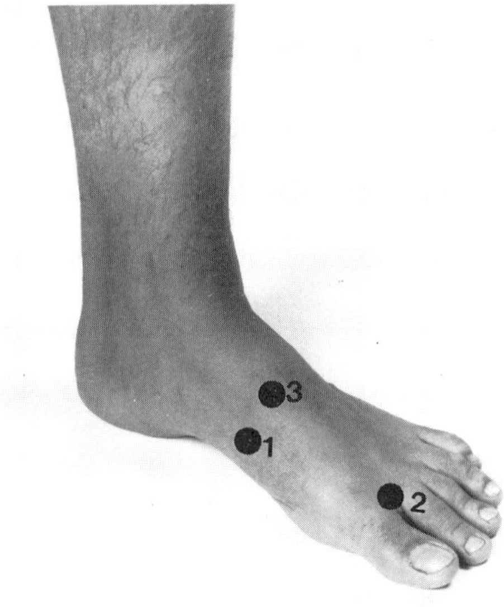


**Point 1**
(P. 4) Left and right
Located on the medial surface of the foot, slightly below the proximal end of the 1st metatarsal bone.

**Point 2**
(Liv. 2) Left and right
Situated on the upper margin of the web between the large toe and the second toe.

**Point 3**
(Liv. 3) Left and right
Located on the lateral surface of the 1st metatarsal bone at the proximal end.

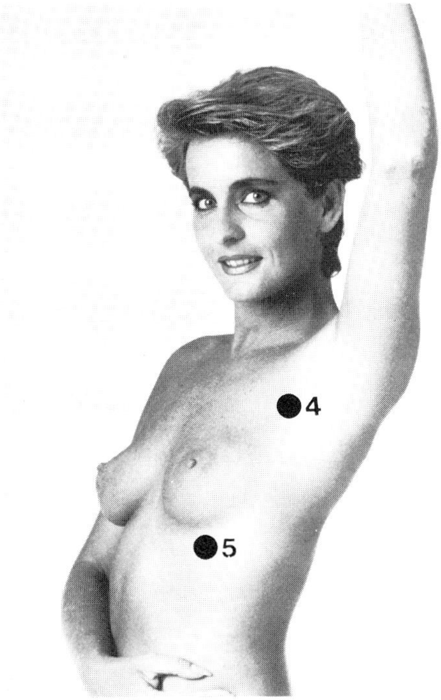


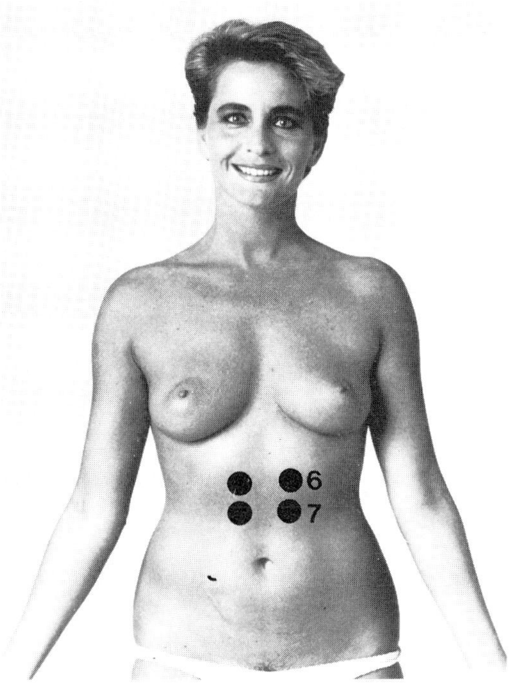


**Point 4**
(G.B. 23) Left and right
Located in the 4th intercostal space, 1 fingerbreadth away from the inner axillary fold line.

**Point 5**
(G.B. 24) Left and right
Located in the 5th intercostal space on the front axillary line (according to Bachmann).

**Point 6**
(St. 21) Left and right
Situated two fingerbreadths offset from the midline, on the same level as the midpoint between the navel and the tip of the xiphoid.

**Point 7**
(St. 22) Left and right
Located in the angle of the 8th intercostal space, approx. 1 fingerbreadth beneath the above described points and 2 fingerbreadths away from the midline of the body.

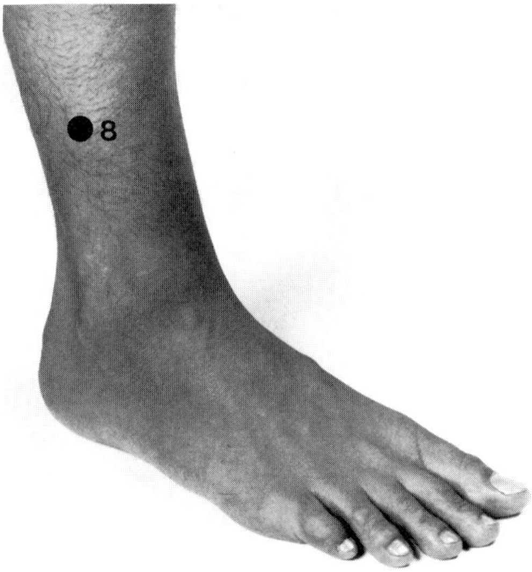


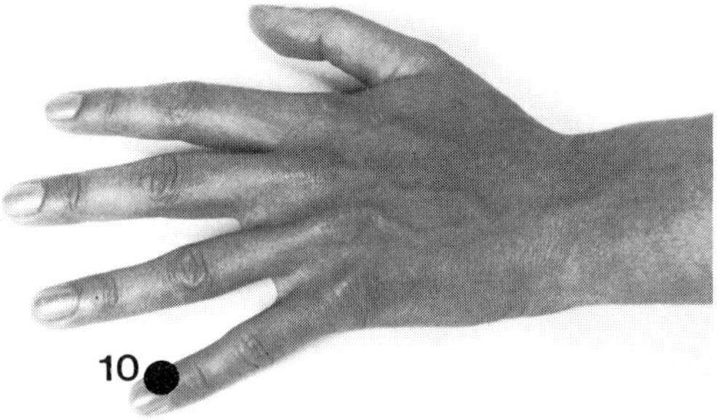


**Point 10**
(H. 9) Left and right
Situated at the medial angle of the nailbed of the small finger, 2 mm diagonally offset.

**Point 8**
(G.B. 38) Left and right
On the lateral front surface of the calf bone, approx. 5 fingerbreadths above the lateral malleolus.

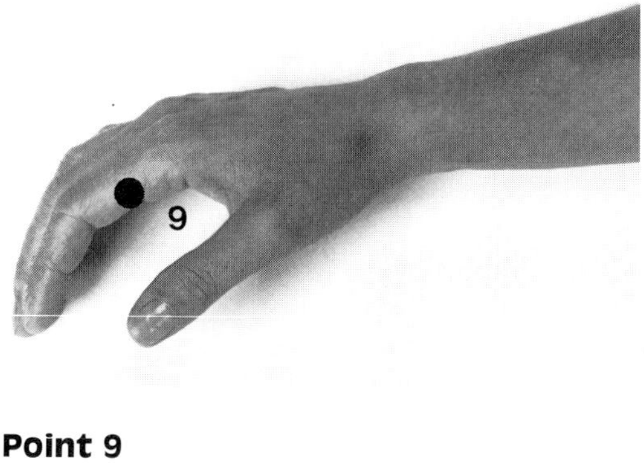


**Point 9**
(S.I. 2) Left and right
Located on the lateral surface of the index finger, approx. 1 fingerbreadth away from the basal joint of the index finger.

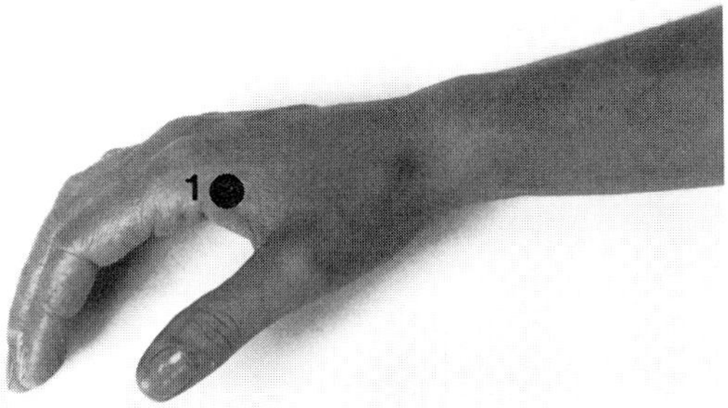


**Point 1**
(S.I. 3) Left and right
Situated above the basal joint of the index finger on the lateral surface, in a small hollow formed by making a fist.

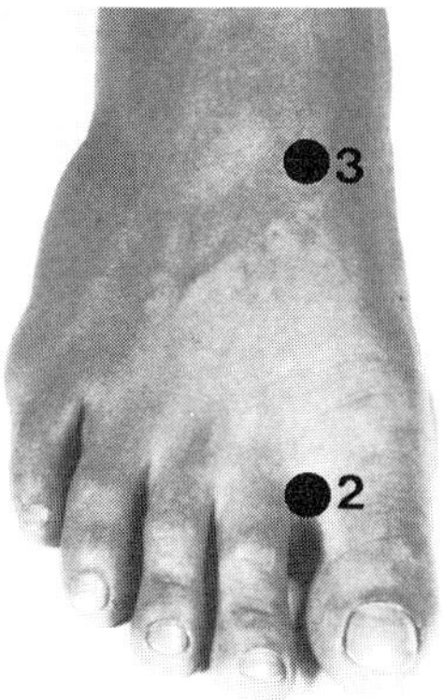


**Point 2**
(Liv. 2) Left and right
Located on the upper margin of the web between the 1st and 2nd toe.

**Point 3**
(Liv. 3) Left and right
Located on the lateral side of the 1st metatarsal bone at the proximal end.

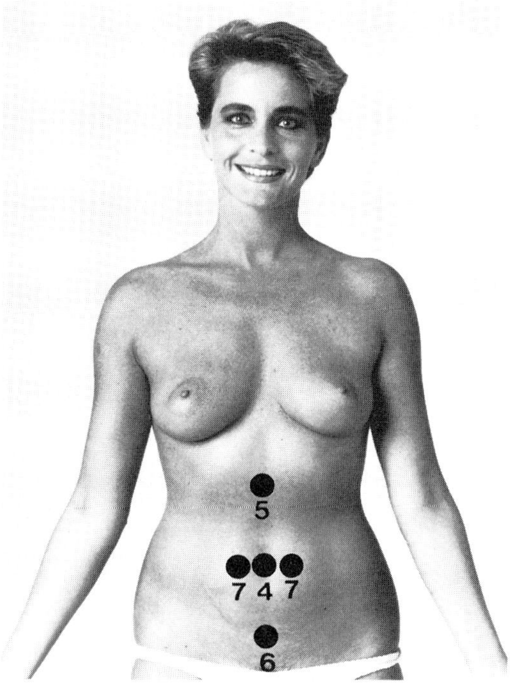


**Point 4**
(C.V. 8)
Situated exactly in the middle of the navel.

**Point 5**
(C.V. 13)
Located on the midline of the body, 1 fingerbreadth above the midpoint between the tip of the xiphoid and the navel (C.V. 12).

**Point 6**
(C.V. 4)
Situated on the midline of the body, at the beginning of the lower third of the section between navel and pubic bone.

**Point 7**
(St. 25) Left and right
Located 2 fingerbreadths laterally offset from the navel.

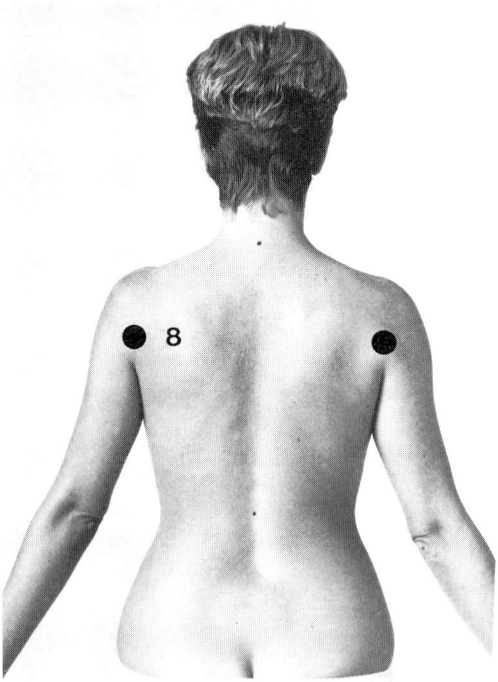


**Point 8**
(S.I. 9) Left and right
Located 2 fingerbreadths above the axillary fold.

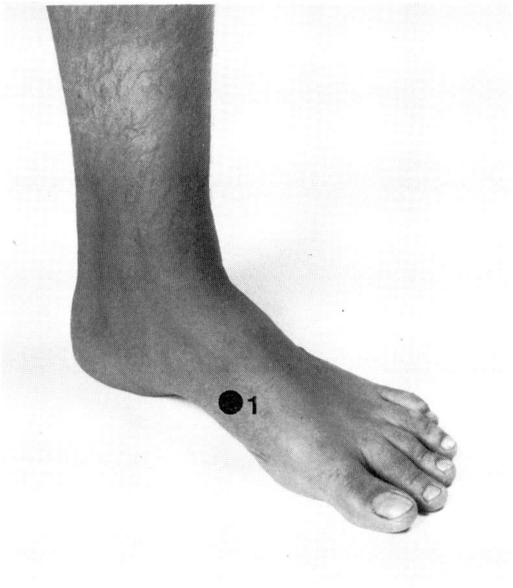


**Point 1**
(P.) Left and right
Located on the medial surface of the foot, slightly beyond the distal end of the 1st metatarsal bone.

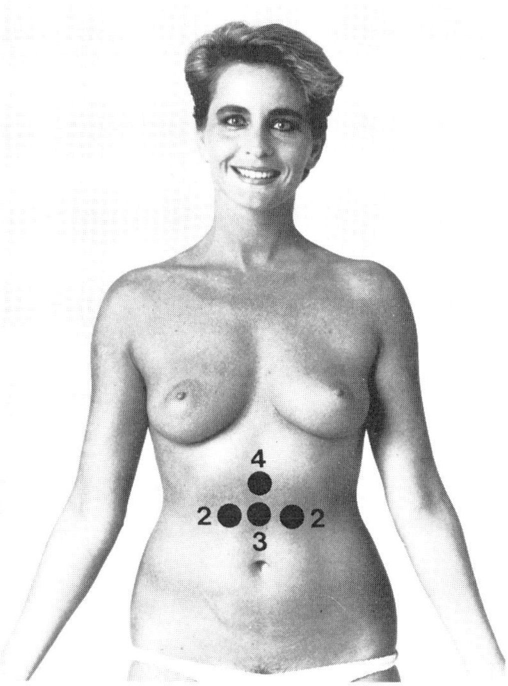


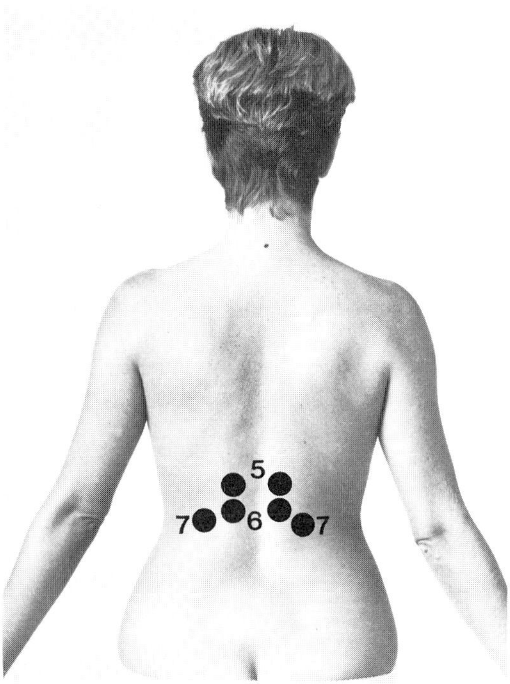


**Point 2**
(St. 21) Left and right
Situated 2 fingerbreadths away from the midline, at the same level as the midpoint between the tip of the xiphoid and the navel.

**Point 3**
(C.V. 12)
Located on the midline at the midpoint between the tip of the xiphoid and the navel.

**Point 4**
(C.V. 13)
Located 1 fingerbreadth above the midpoint between the tip of the xiphoid and the navel (C.V. 12).

**Point 5**
(U.B. 20) Left and right
Situated in the 11th intercostal space, 2 fingerbreadths offset from the midline of the body.

**Point 6**
(U.B. 21) Left and right
Located in the 12th intercostal space, 2 fingerbreadths offset from the midline of the body.

**Point 7**
(U.B. 45) Left and right
Situated approx. a hand's breadth away from the midline on level with the 12th thoracic vertebra.

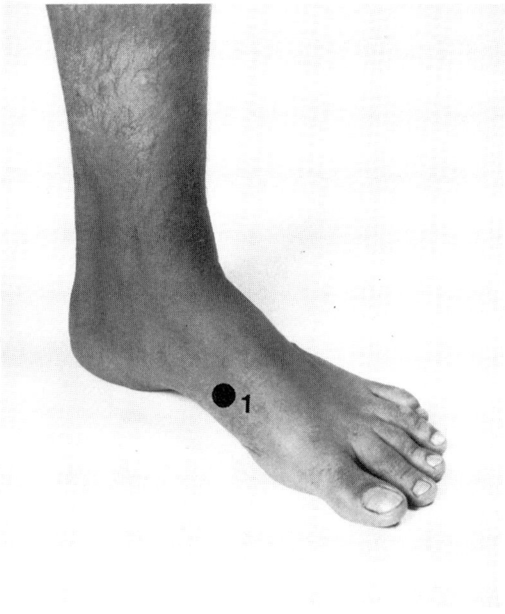


**Point 1**

(P. 4) Left and right

Located on the medial surface of the foot, slightly below the proximal end of the 1st metatarsal bone.

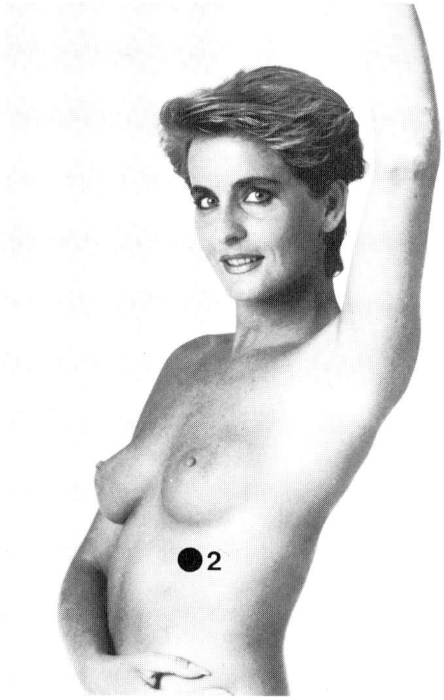


**Point 2**

(G.B. 24) Left and right)

Situated in the 5th intercostal space on the front axillary line (according to Bachmann).

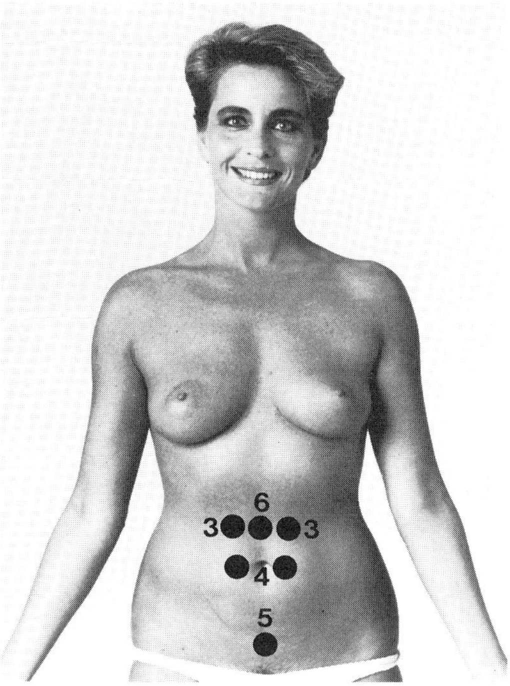


**Point 3**
(St. 21) Left and right
Located 2 fingerbreadths away from the midline, on level with the midpoint between the tip of the xiphoid and the navel.

**Point 4**
(St. 25) Left and right
Situated 2 fingerbreadths offset from the middle of the navel.

**Point 5**
(C.V. 4)
Situated on the midline of the body, at the beginning of the lower third of the section between navel and pubic bone.

**Point 6**
(C.V. 12)
Located at the midpoint between the tip of the xiphoid and the navel, on the midline.

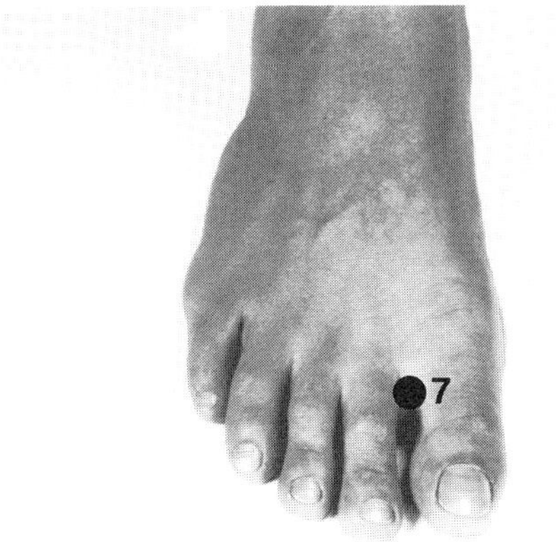


**Point 7**
(Liv. 2) Left and right
Located on the upper margin of the web between the 1st and 2nd toe.

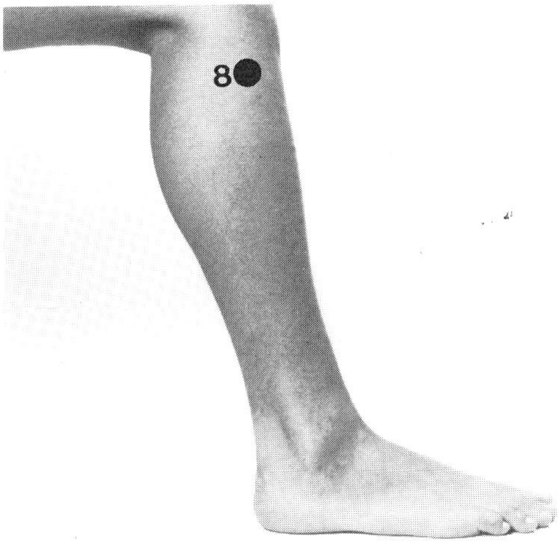


**Point 8**
(St.36) Left and right
Located on the lateral, anterior surface of the lower leg, on the middle of the shin bone three fingerbreadths below the knee. This point can also be determined by placing the palm of the hand on the knee – the tip of the middle finger aims at the point.

# First-Aid Treatment with the Acu-Impulsor

1. Ear Points
2. Hand Acupuncture
3. Head Points

How often does it happen that we suddenly experience pain or unpleasant symptoms while travelling or on holiday. If there is no doctor or health practitioner available, this can be a most annoying experience indeed. Whether headaches, complaints of the spine or the joints, stomachache or other condition treatment with the acu-impulsor will be able to bring quick relief in many cases. In many instances a considerable amount of time may pass until such conditions can be properly diagnosed. Therefore this type of acu-impulsor treatment can be regarded as a kind of first aid. There are three zones of points which are particularly suited for this purpose, namely the acupuncture points located on the ear, the hands and the points situated on the head.

The system of ear acupuncture presumably has ancient origins. The French physician Nogier is regarded as being the founder of modern ear acupuncture. He has established a system which was initially based on observations made with patients suffering from very serious diseases and which he termed "Auriculo-Therapy". In Germany it was Niels Krack, M.D., a student of Nogier, who in turn made a number of developments of his own and published a topography of the ear points with a special numerical coding. My colleague Günter Lange, from Kassel, West Germany, himself a student of Niels Krack, has been compiling in-depth information on the individual schools of acupuncture for many years now and has recently published a summary of his work as a book. His reputation as one of the foremost practitioners for auricular therapy is also founded on his numerous discoveries in this area.

There can be no doubt as to the fact that the acupuncture points of the ear are capable of transmitting therapeutic resonance impulses via the brain to the disordered sectors of the body. Treatment with the acu-impulsor is not intended to replace auricular acupuncture. However it is of paramount importance to be able to do something immediately for painful conditions. In such cases the use of the handy acu-impulsor is legitimate and simple. In the following I have numbered the most important points for treating the spine and joints. These suggestions are also based on the experience I have gained in the use of the acu-impulsor to date. For the sake of simplicity I have numbered the points in the ear from 1 to 23.

Ear point indications:
Nos. 1, 2 and 3: Inflammation
Nos. 4 and 5: Head

| | |
|---|---|
| Nr. 6: Cervical spine | Nr. 7: Neck |
| Nr. 8: Collar bone | Nr. 9: Shoulder joints |
| Nr. 10: Thoracic spine | Nr. 11: Shoulder |
| Nr. 12: Lumbar spine | Nr. 13: Elbow |
| Nr. 14: Buttocks | Nr. 15: Sciatica |
| Nr. 16: Pain point | Nr. 17: Wrist |
| Nr. 18: Finger | Nr. 19: Hip joint |
| Nr. 20: Knee joint | Nr. 21: Ankle |
| Nr. 22: Heel | Nr. 23: Toes |

Points Nr. 1, 2 and 3 are the first points treated in all conditions of pain and are followed by those points related to the affected area.

Example: Shoulder complaints
Points 1, 2 and 3 are given 10 impulses each. Then treat point 11, point 6 and point 7 with 10 impulses each, adhering to this sequence.

Example 2: Knee complaints
Treat point nos. 1, 2 and 3 first and subsequently point 19, applying 10 impulses each. Points 1, 2 and 3 must always be treated before turning to the point related to the painful area.

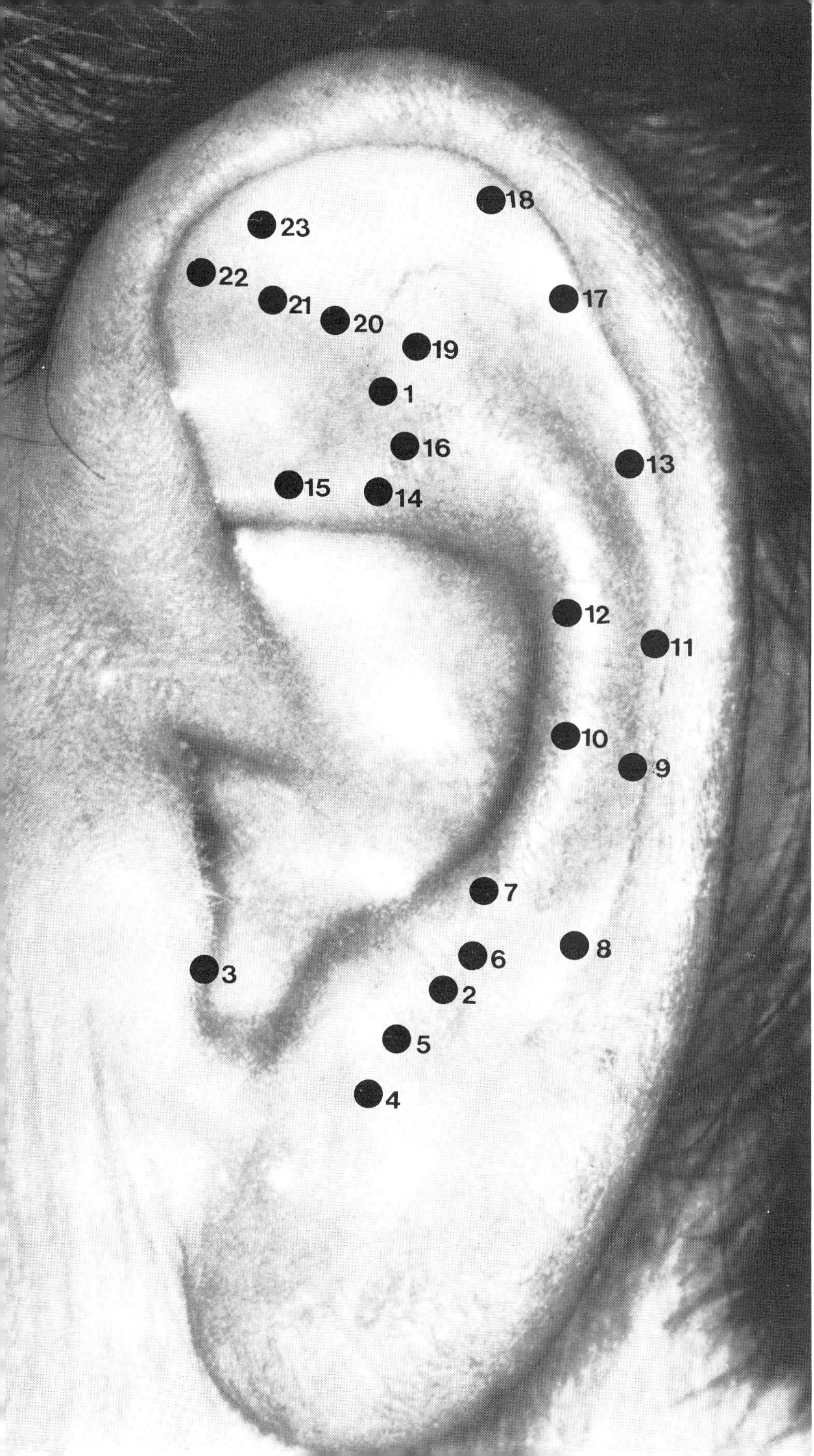
18
23
22
17
21
20
19
1
16
13
15
14
12
11
10
9
7
8
6
3
2
5
4

The second method for fast pain relief is via the hand acupuncture system. The points situated there are related to the individual organs and are easy to find and treat.

The hand points are so-called reflex points, just like the ear points and the zones on the foot. They are connected to the network of the meridians and are presumably capable of transmitting reflexes directly to the cerebral control systems where resonance forces which restore balance to the disordered organs and systems are then released.

Point 1: Pain of the lumbar spine
Point 2: Pain of the lumbar spine
Point 3: Pain caused by injury or rheumatic pain of the wrist
Point 4: Pain in the region of the nose
Point 5: Headache
Point 6: Eye point, pain of the eyes, inflammations, pain caused by glaucoma
Point 7: Stiffness of the shoulders, shoulder pain
Point 8: Pain of the cervical spine
Point 9: Toothache, pain and inflammation of the tonsils, pain of the larynx, trigeminal neuralgia
Point 10: Pain of the buttocks, sciatica, pain of the hip joint
Point 11: Pain after spinal operations, pain of the lumbar spine, congested nose
Point 12: Pain in the region of the anus and fissures
Point 13: Pain at the vertex
Point 14: Frontal headaches, cramps in the entire abdomen
Point 15: Occipital pain, pain of the arms, pain in the region of the cheeks, tonsillitis
Point 16: Migraine, pain caused by gallbladder colic, pain in the thorax, pain in the left and right upper abdomen
Point 17: Intercostal neuralgias, diarrhea, pain caused by herpes zoster
Point 18: Pain and rheumatism of the ankle joints
Point 19: Nose bleeding

Point 20: Pain in the region of the heel
Point 21: Nervous headache, bronchitis, asthma
Point 22: Hysteria
Point 23: Hyperhidrosis – excessive sweating on the hands, feet and in the armpits
Point 24: Asthma, bronchitis, cough
Point 25: Nervous heart complaints
Point 26: Ulcers of the mucous membranes of the oral cavity
Point 27: Bed wetting
Point 28: Bed wetting
Point 29: Gastric and duodenal ulcers, digestive disorders, gastritis

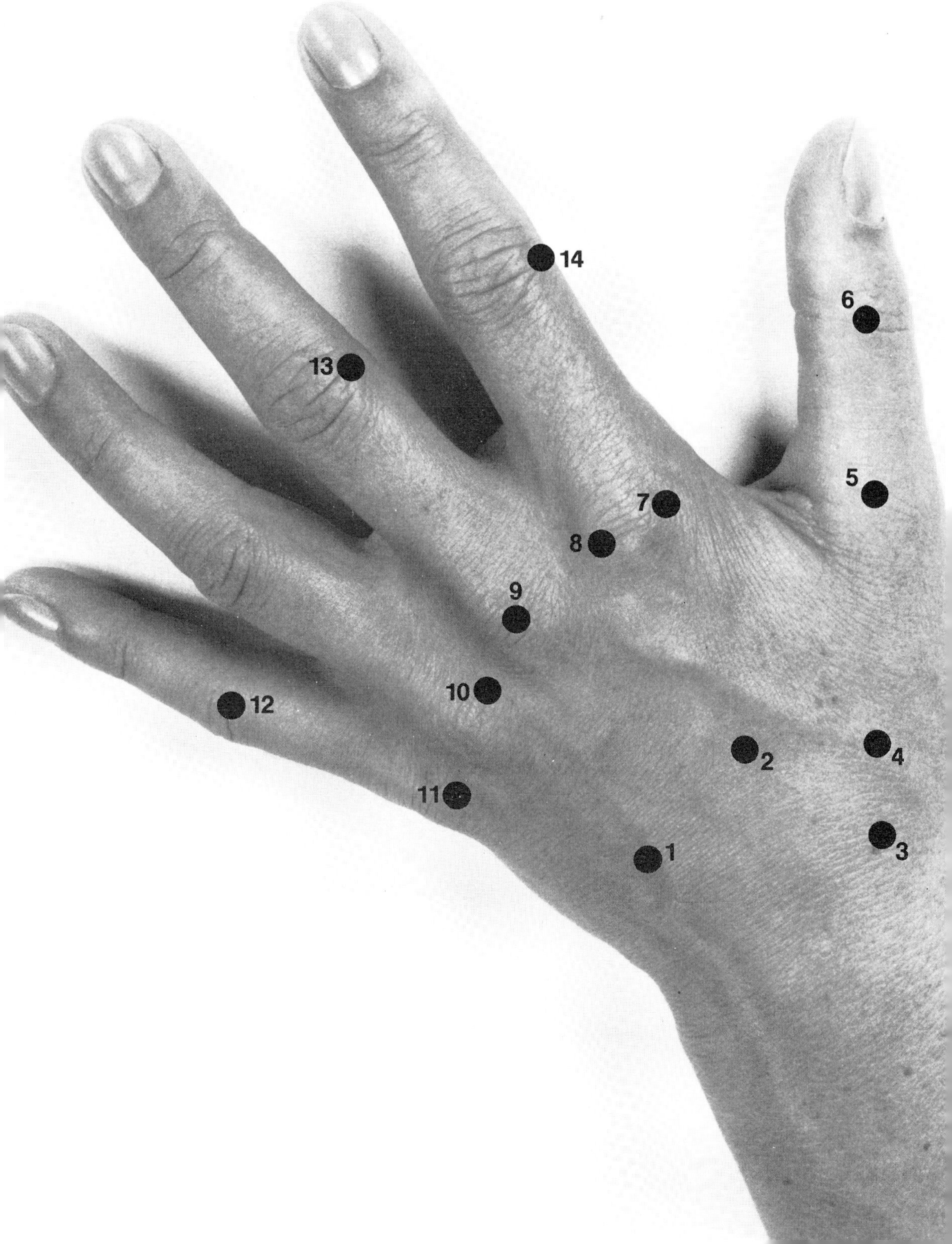

1
2
3
4
5
6
7
8
9
10
11
12
13
14

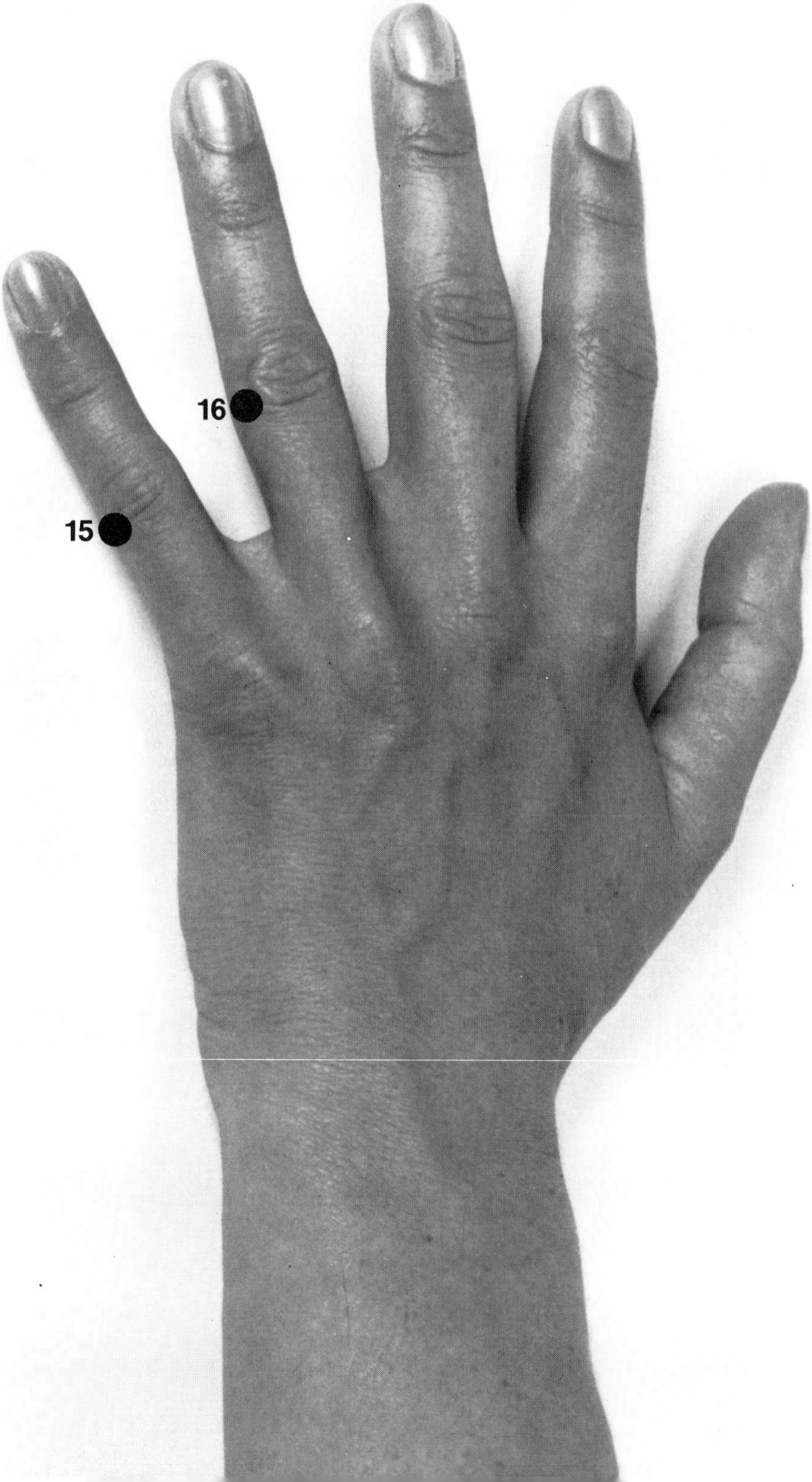
16
15

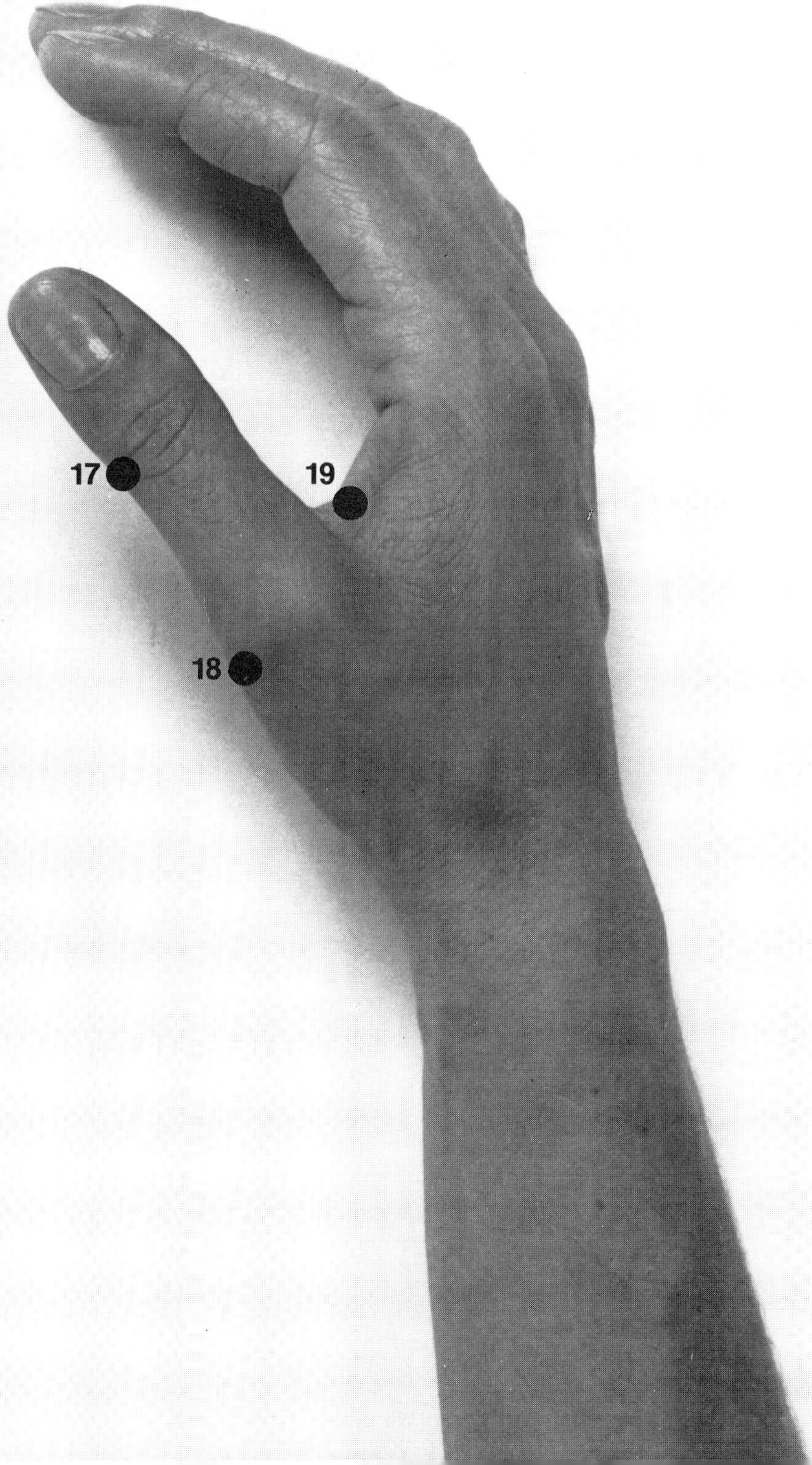
17
19
18

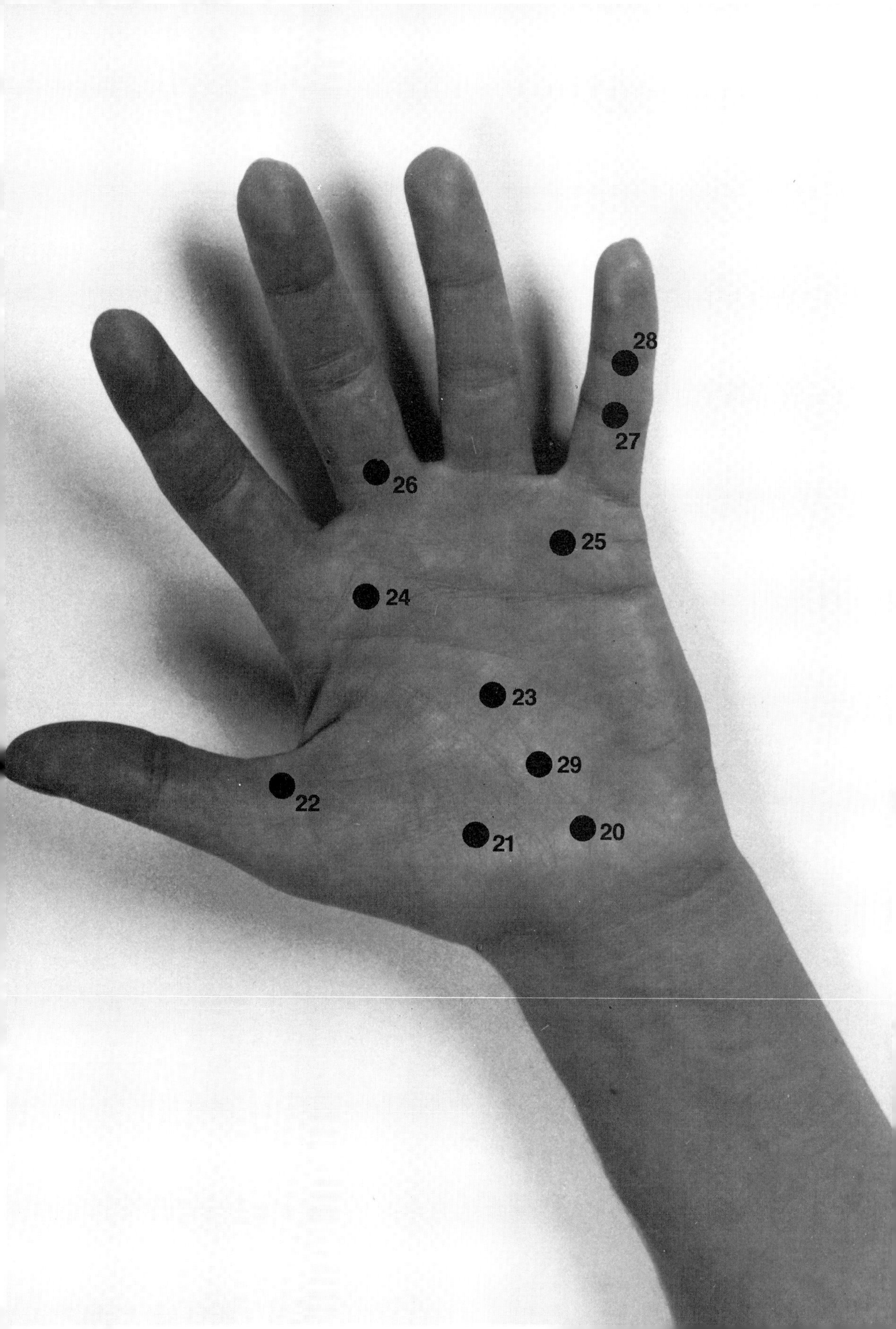
28
27
26
25
24
23
29
22
21
20

A third method of treating conditions of acute pain consists of the acu-impulsor treatment of individual points located on the head. During the course of my work with energy phenomena, I discovered relays which are situated in seven places on the body and which, in my opinion, hold a key position in terms of energetic information. I have termed these centers "energetic transmitter relays". These relays are similar to the ripples that spread out when a stone hits a pool of water. On each of these concentric rings, which can be exactly localized, there are highly effective points which are often identical with classical acupuncture points, yet which show a completely different scope of action when treated accordingly.
The points situated on the head have been known for a considerable time and have been used in physio-energetics for diagnostic purposes. For many years I have been employing these points for test therapy in pain conditions of all kinds. I was astonished to find that these points are located on the concentric rings of the energetic transmitter relays I had discovered. These points on the head are all directly linked with the cerebral control organs, which may explain the often instantaneous effects achieved in the treatment of pain. I have numbered the points as follows.

The points 1–6 on the head can all be employed in conditions of pain, regardless of the region of the body affected. Examine all points and treat only those which have been found to be painful with the acu-impulsor.

Names of the points 1–6:

Point 1: Thalamus
Point 2: Hypothalamus
Point 3: Limbic System
Point 4: Epiphysis
Point 5: Hypophysis
Point 6: Corpus callosum

Carry out treatment as follows:
Use the rod which has been provided along with the acu-impulsor to examine the areas where the specified points are located. The exact point is always more painful than the surrounding area. In the case of bilateral points always opt for the more sensitive one. In most cases, the treatment of three points is enough to achieve immediate amelioration. The sensitive points are given 15 impulses each – repeat after 15 minutes as required.

These three methods for treating pain can also be combined. It is amazing how quickly the treatment of the points calls forth resonance forces which ameliorate or dispel pain altogether.

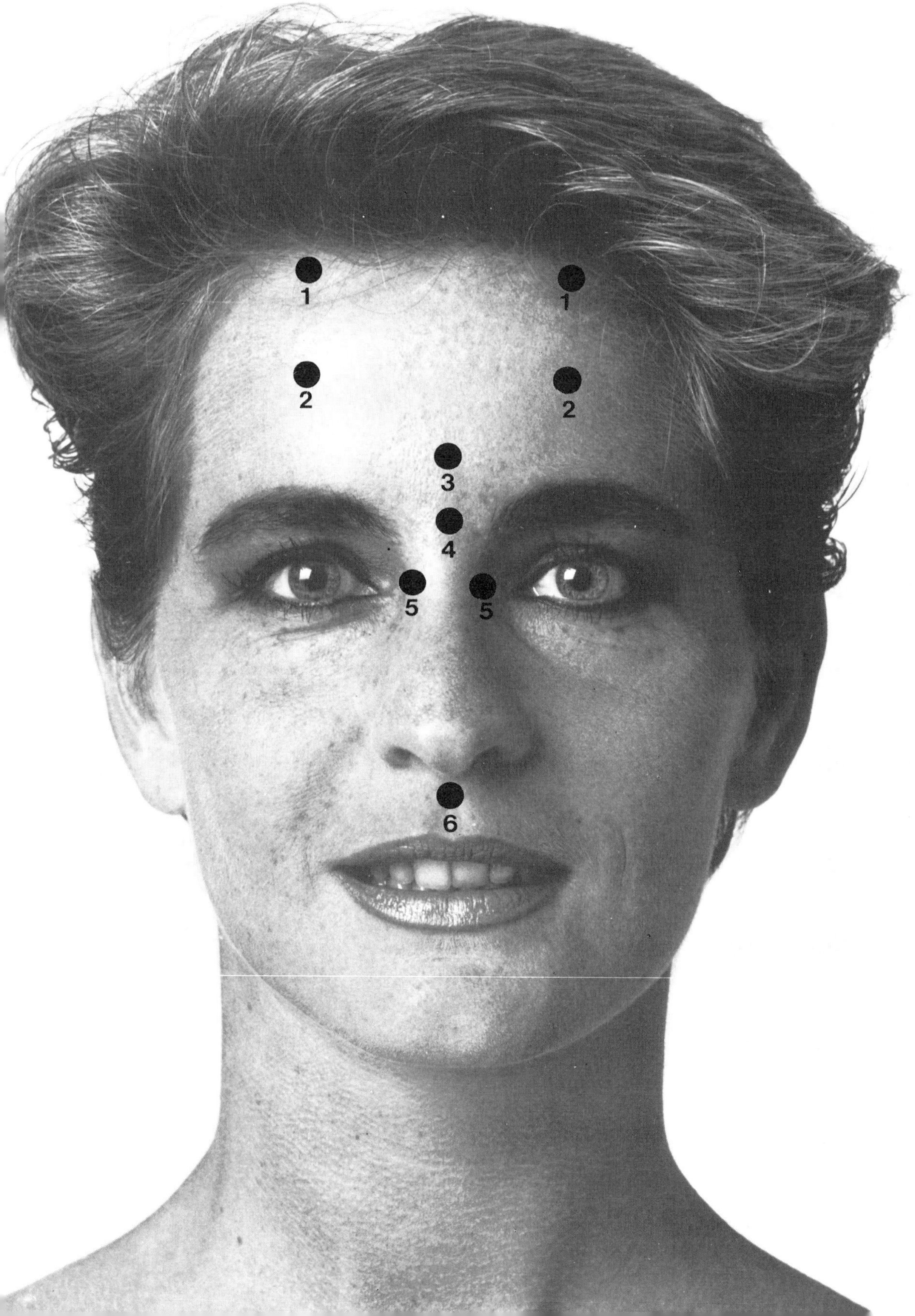
1
1
2
2
3
4
5
5
6

# Allergies and Skin Diseases

1. General Allergy Points
2. Asthma I
3. Asthma II
4. Eczema
5. Hay Fever
6. Acute Hay Fever
7. Acne

The drastic increase in allergies over the past years is an alarming development involving many children. Particularly skin allergies, hay fever, asthma and food allergies are on the rise and pose serious problems for the persons affected. According to the standpoint of natural therapeutics, these are symptoms pointing to an immune system which is no longer functioning properly. A healthy immune system is generally capable of dealing with a wide range of allergy-causing substances without producing those dreaded symptoms which in some cases can develop into potentially fatal conditions.

In this context, it is also particularly important to determine which substances are causing the given allergy. In the case of asthma, we may be dealing with a number of contributing factors which must be thoroughly diagnosed. One must differentiate between those types of asthma which are based on organic disorders of the respiratory organs, those which are caused by heart disorders and finally the spastic (vegetative) and allergic asthma forms. Persons suffering from hay fever are allergic to a number of different types of pollen from flowering grasses and trees.

We are confronted with a wide range of causes which cannot all be dealt with here.

The treatment of allergies is carried out as follows:

**1. Asthma**

1. Control I
2. Allergy points
3. Asthma I
4. Asthma II

Repeat the treatment of points 1 - 4 and alternate daily.

**2. Hay Fever**

Treat the following combinations:

1. Lymph treatment
2. Allergy points
3. Hay fever points - alternated these combinations daily.

All disorders having an allergic component should also be treated intermediately with the combinations for intestinal and metabolic functioning.

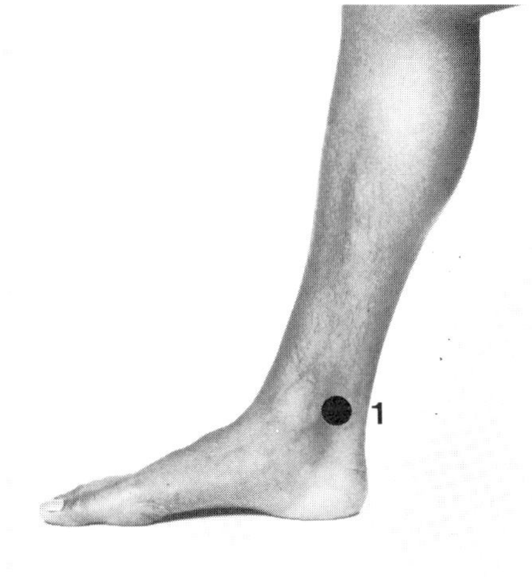


**Point 1**
(K. 3) Left and right
Located 1 fingerbreadth behind the medial ankle bone, approx. in the middle between malleolus and the achilles tendon.

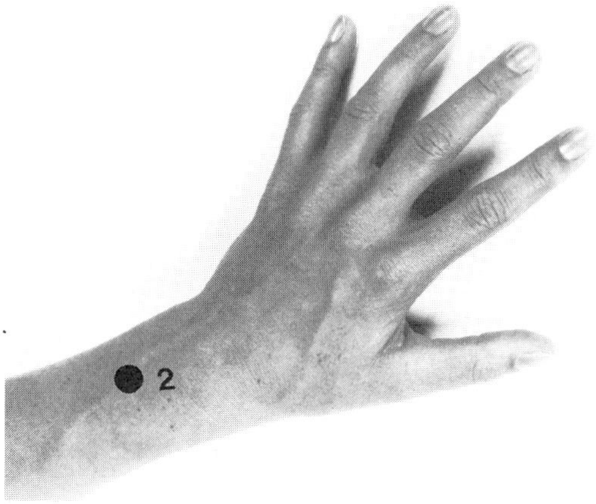


**Point 2**
(T.H. 5) Left and right
Located approx. 2½ fingerbreadths above the wrist fold between ulna and radius.

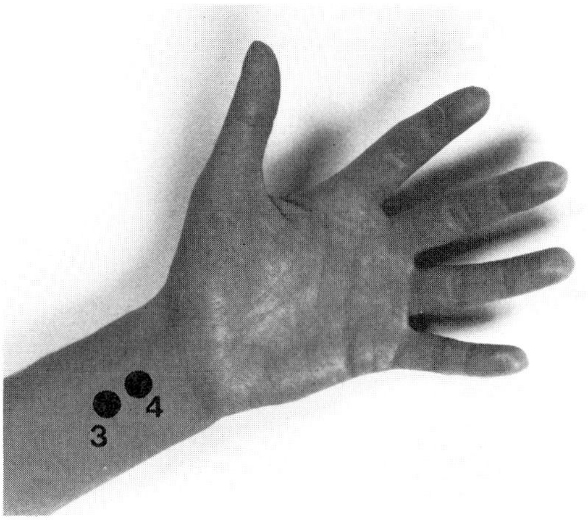


**Point 3**
(C.V. 5) Left and right
Situated approx. 4 fingerbreadths above the first wrist fold in the middle of the medial surface of the forearm.

**Point 4**
(C. 6) Left and right
Located approximately 3 fingerbreadths above the first wrist fold in the middle of the medial surface of the forearm.

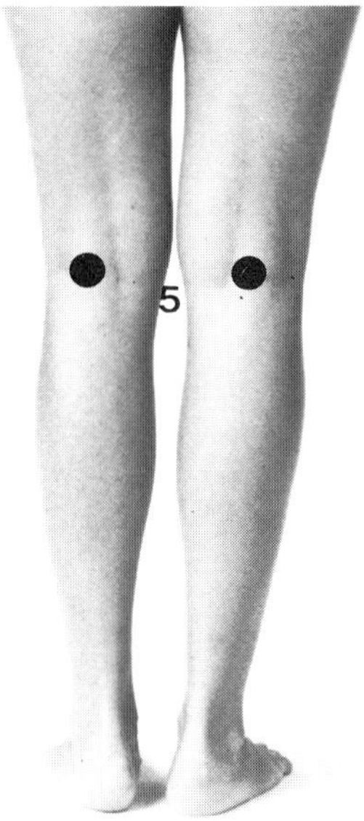


**Point 5**
(U.B. 54) Left and right
Located in the middle of the hollow of the knee.

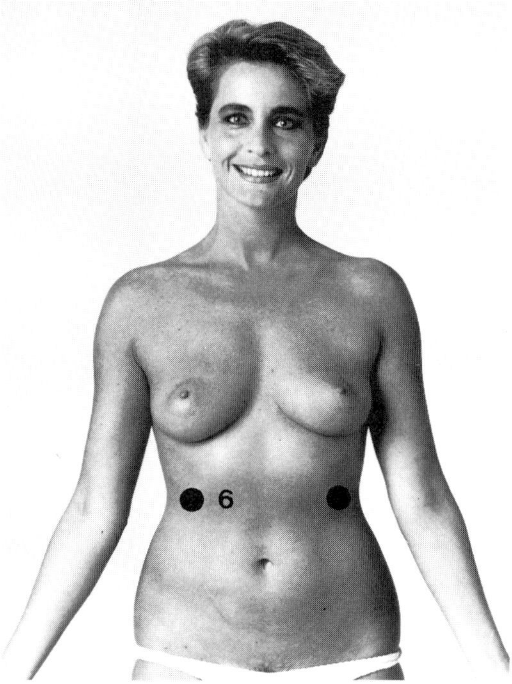


**Point 6**
(Liv. 13) Left and right
Situated on the llth rib, slightly offset from the medial end.

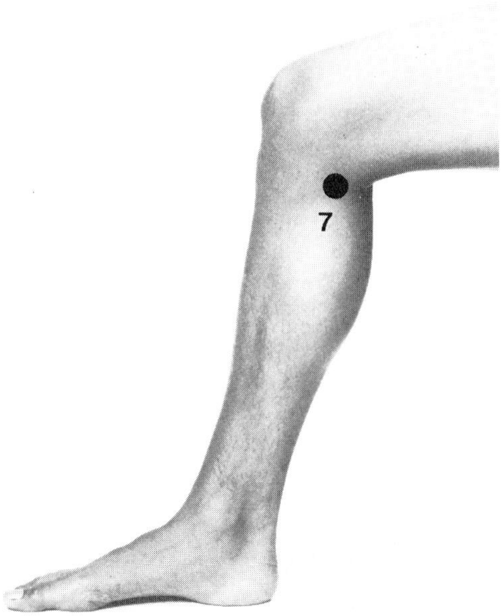


**Point 7**
(Liv. 8) Left and right
Located on the posterior, medial surface of the knee, on the gap of the joint, directly behind the tendon which can be felt there.

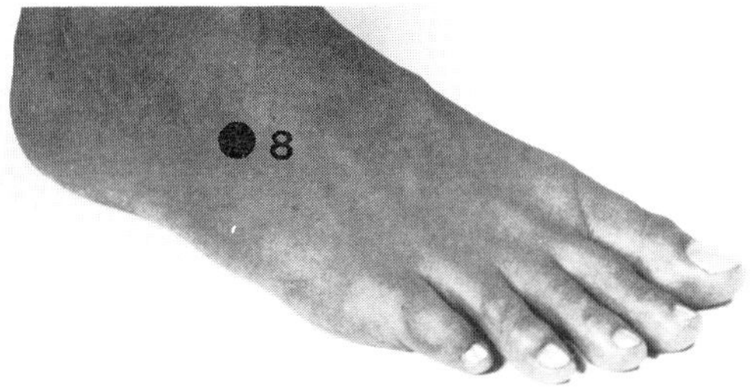


**Point 8**
(G.B. 41) Left and right
Situated on the back of the foot between the 4th and 5th metatarsal bones at their proximal end.

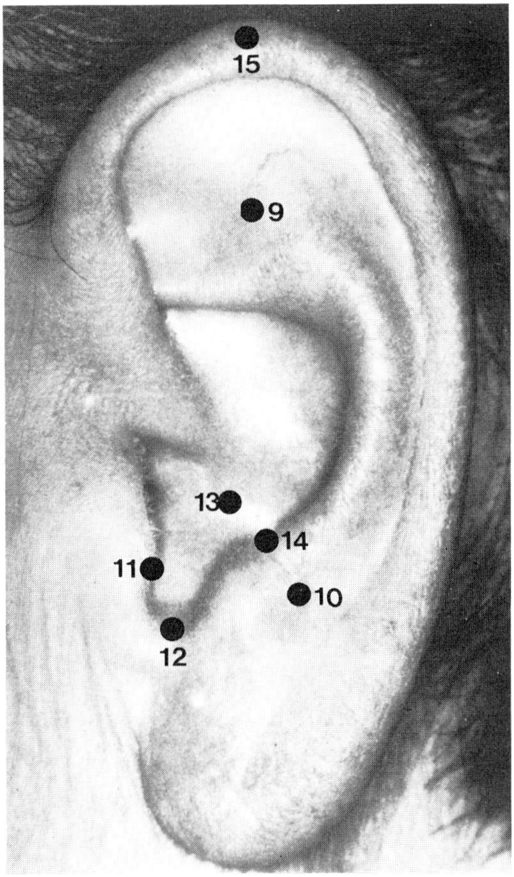


**Point 9:** Ear point
**Point 10:** Ear point
**Point 11:** Ear point
**Point 12:** Ear point
**Point 13:** Ear point
**Point 14:** Ear point
**Point 15:** Ear point

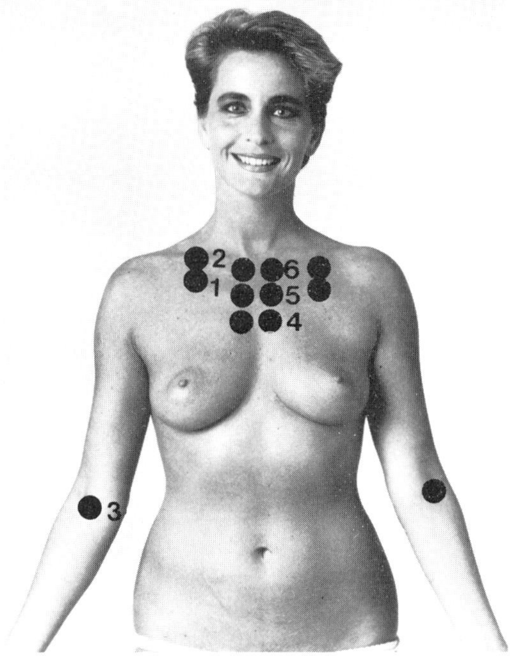


**Point 1**
(L. 1) Left and right
This point is located approximately 1 fingerbreadth below the lower margin of the collar bone in the middle of the 1st intercostal space.

**Point 2**
(L. 2) Left and right
Located exactly above the first lung point, on the lower margin of the collar bone.

**Point 3**
(L. 5) Left and right
When the forearm is flexed this point will be found on the medial surface of the tendon of the biceps muscle.

**Point 4**
(K. 25) Left and right
Located in the second intercostal space directly next to the sternum, approximately 2 fingerbreadths offset from the midline of the body.

**Point 5**
(K. 26) Left and right
Located in the 1st intercostal space, directly next to the sternum, 2 fingerbreadths offset from the midline.

**Point 6**
(K. 27) Left and right
Located below the conjunction of collar bone and sternum.

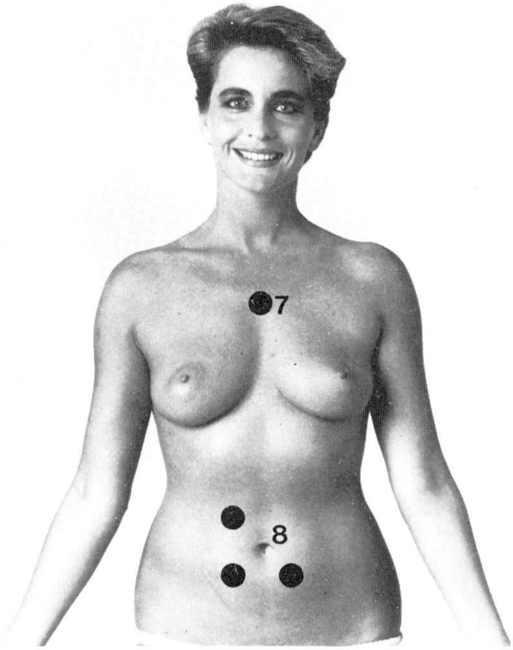


**Point 7**
(C.V. 17)
Located on the midline on the sternum, on level with the 4th intercostal space.

**Point 8**
(Aggressive zones)
Draw two lines intersecting the navel at a 45 degree angle. The first point is to the left below the navel, the second point is at the right below the navel and the third to the right above the navel – all points are 2 fingerbreadths offset from the navel.

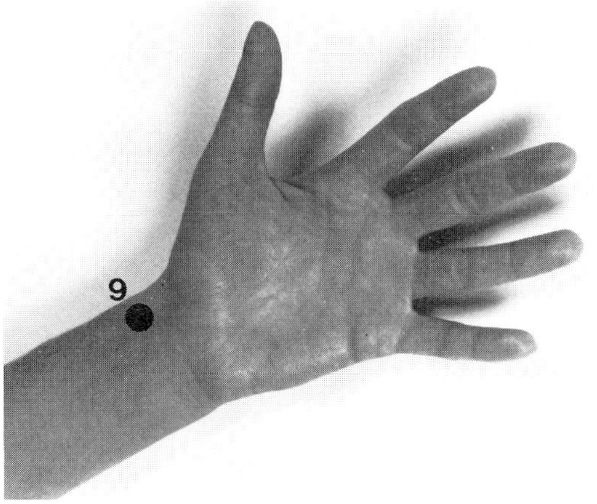


**Point 9**
(L. 7) Left and right
Located approx. 2 fingerbreadths offset from the first wrist fold in the so-called radial groove.

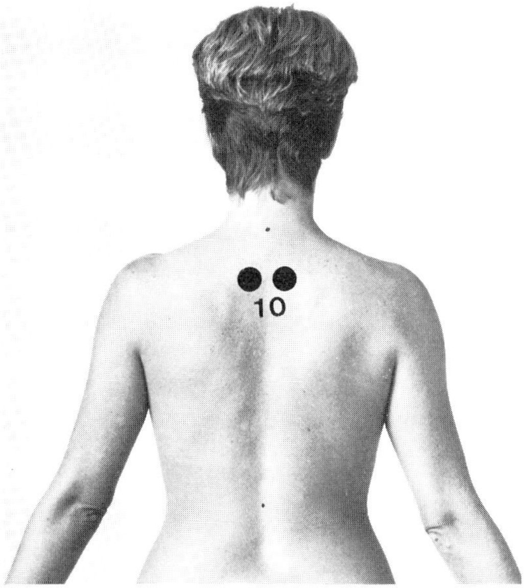


**Point 10**
(U.B. 13) Left and right
Situated in the 3rd intercostal space 2 fingerbreadths away from the midline.

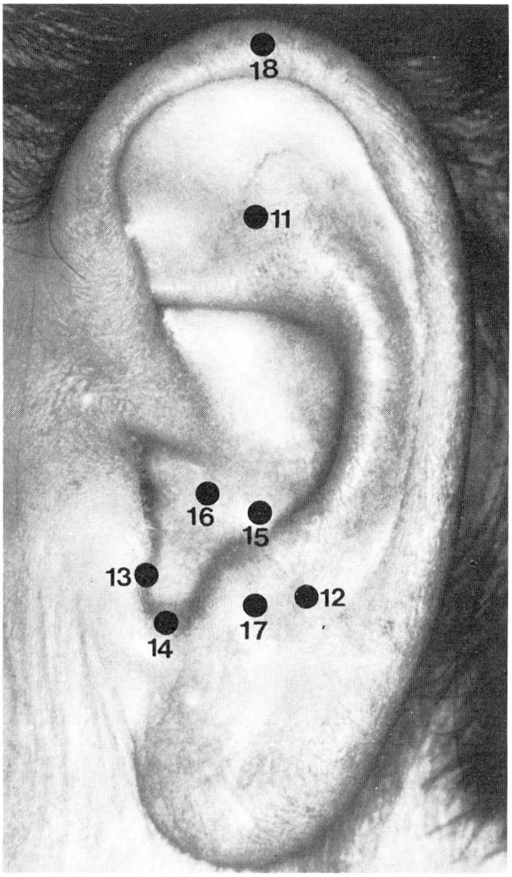


**Point 11:** Ear point
**Point 12:** Ear point
**Point 13:** Ear point
**Point 14:** Ear point
**Point 15:** Ear point
**Point 16:** Ear point
**Point 17:** Ear point
**Point 18:** Ear point

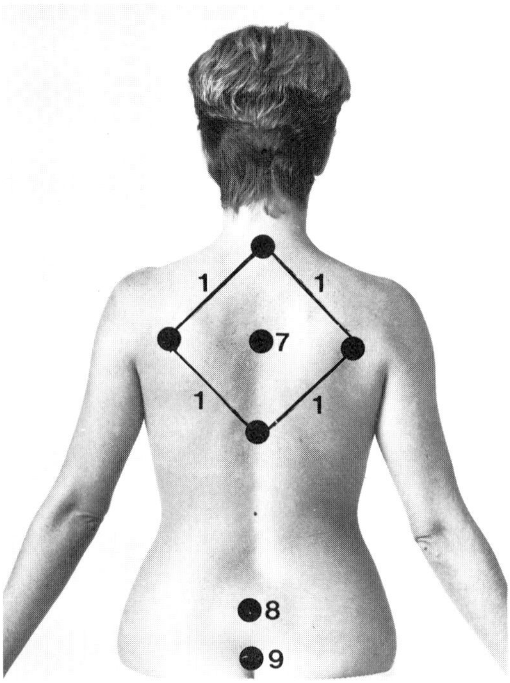


**Point 1**
(Lymph rhombus)
This rhombus is formed by the following 4 acupuncture points –

S.I. 11 – left and right
This point is located in the middle of the shoulder blade, below a crest which can be felt there.

G.V. 13
This point is situated directly on the tip of the spinal process of the 7 cervical vertebra.

G.V. 6
This point is located directly on the spinal process of the 11th thoracic vertebra.

**Point 7**
(G.V. point directly opposite C.V. 18)
Located on the midline of the spine, on a horizontal line drawn between the two midpoints of the shoulder blade.

**Point 8**
Situated in the middle of the sacrum.
**Point 9**
Located at the beginning of the anal fold on the midline of the body.

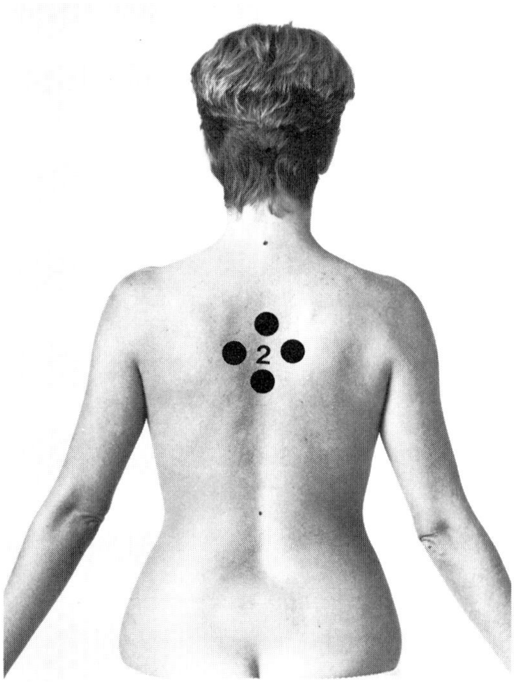


**Point 2**
(Life rhombus)
The rhombus midpoint is located on the midline of the spine, on level with the midpoint of the shoulder blade. The 4 rhombus points are grouped around the central point on the spine at a distance of approx. 2 fingerbreadths.

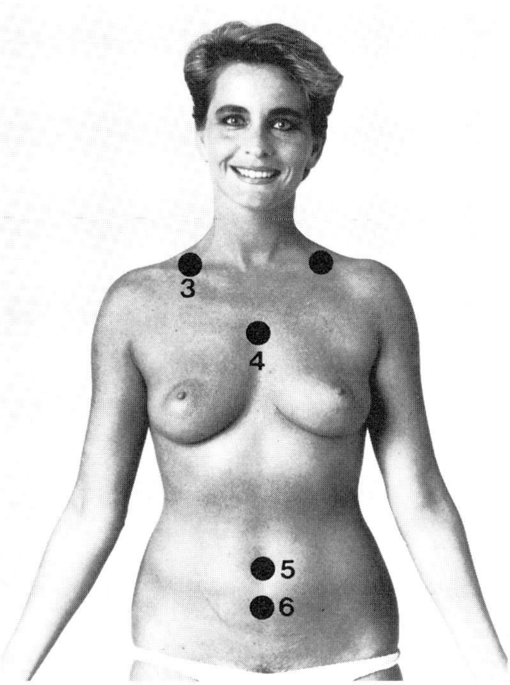


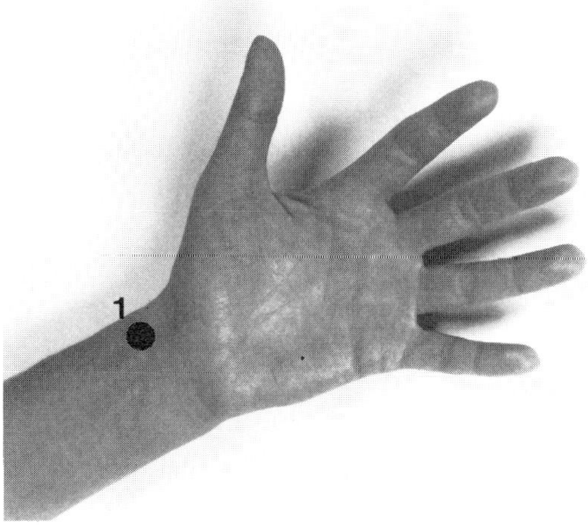


**Point 1**
(L. 7) Left and right
Located approx. 2 fingerbreadths away from the 1st wrist fold in the so-called radial groove.

**Point 3**
(St. 12) Left and right
Located on the mammary line on the upper margin of the collar bone, approx. 4 fingerbreadths offset from the midline of the body.

**Point 4**
(C.V. 18)
Located on the midline on the sternum – on level with the 3rd intercostal space.

**Point 5**
(C.V. 8)
Located exactly in the middle of the navel.

**Point 6**
(C.V. 6)
Situated approx. 2 fingerbreadths below the navel on the midline.

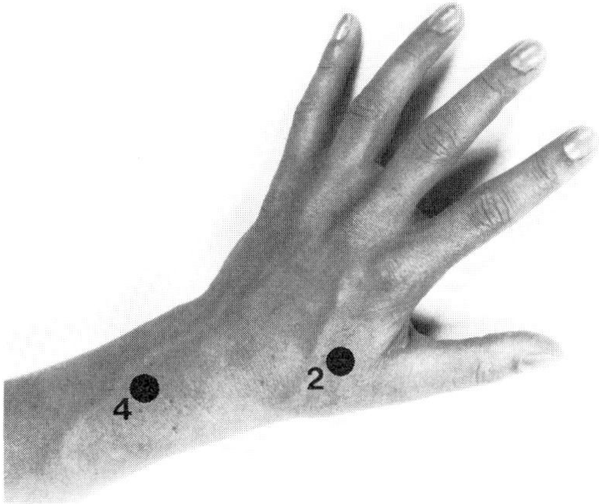


**Point 2** (L.I. 4) Left and right
Located on the medial side of the index finger in the angle formed by the thumb and the index finger.

**Point 4** (T.H. 5) Left and right
Situated approx. 2½ fingerbreadths above the wrist fold in the middle between ulna and radius.

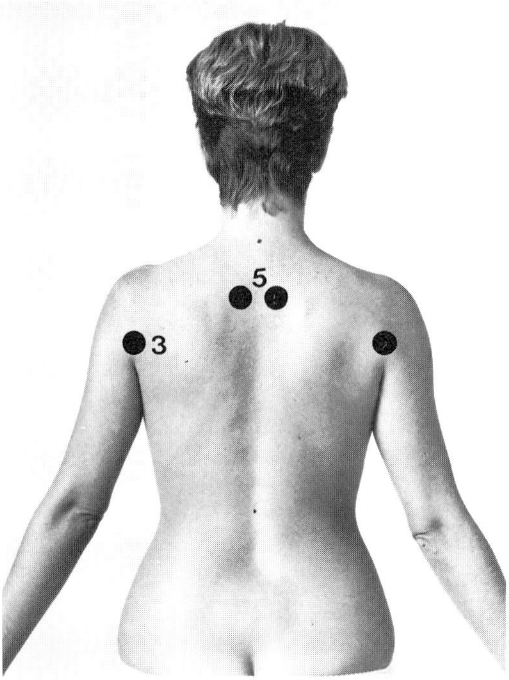


**Point 3**
(S.I. 9) Left and right
Located 2 fingerbreadths above the axillary fold.

**Point 5**
(U.B. 13) Left and right
Located 2 fingerbreadths offset from the midline of the body in the 3rd intercostal space.

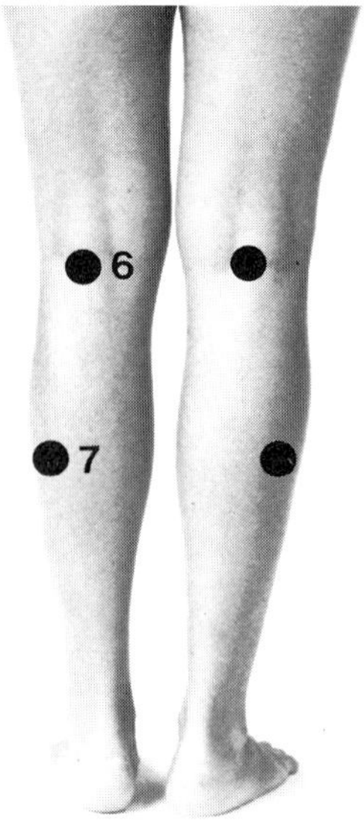


**Point 6**
(U.B. 54) Left and right
Located in the middle of the hollow of the knee.

**Point 7**
(U.B. 58) Left and right
Located in the middle of the ankle on the lateral surface.

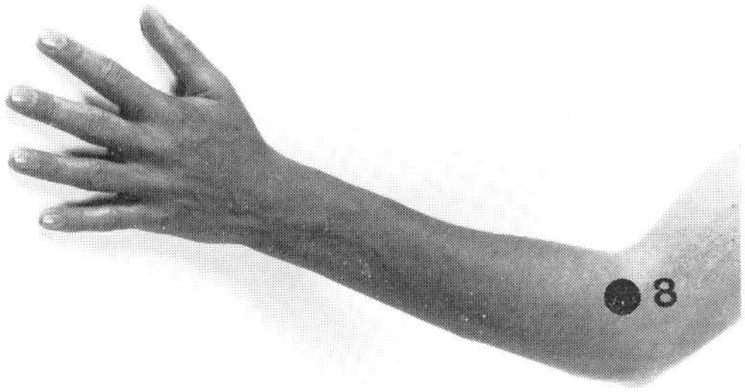


**Point 8**
(S.I. 11) Left and right
Located at the medial end of the upper elbow fold.

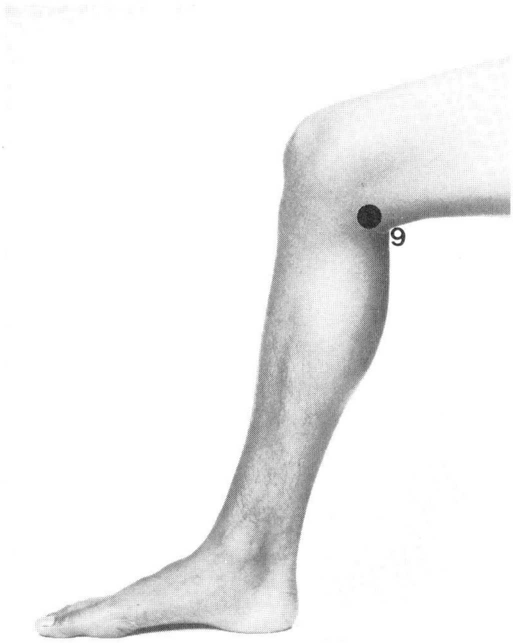


**Point 9**
(Liv. 8) Left and right
Located on the medial surface of the knee on the gap of the knee joint, directly behind the tendon which can be felt there.

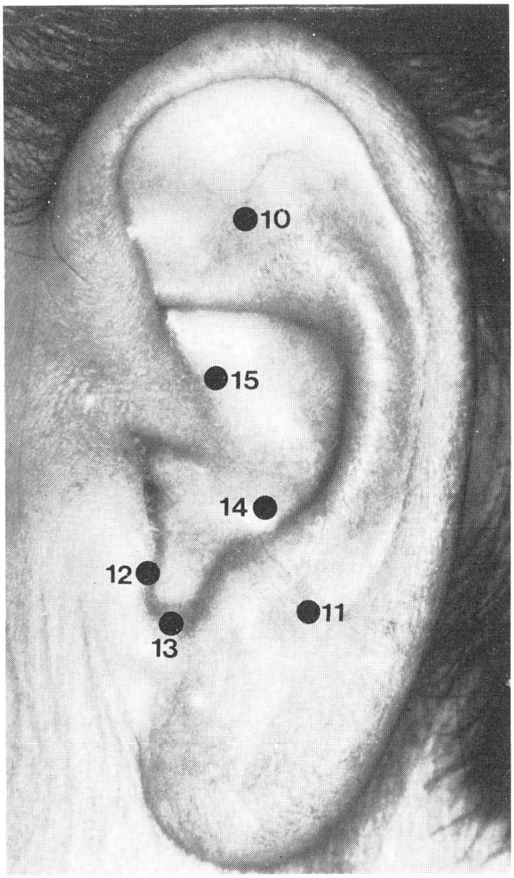


**Point 10:** Ear point
**Point 11:** Ear point
**Point 12:** Ear point
**Point 13:** Ear point
**Point 14:** Ear point
**Point 15:** Ear point

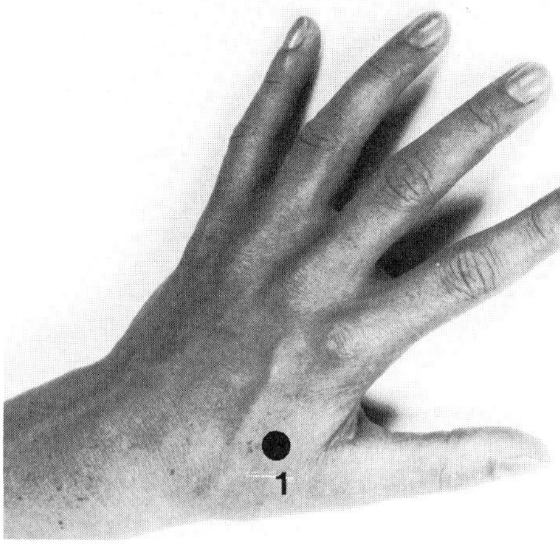


**Point 1**
(S.I. 4) Left and right
Located on the medial surface of the index finger in the angle formed by the thumb and the index finger.

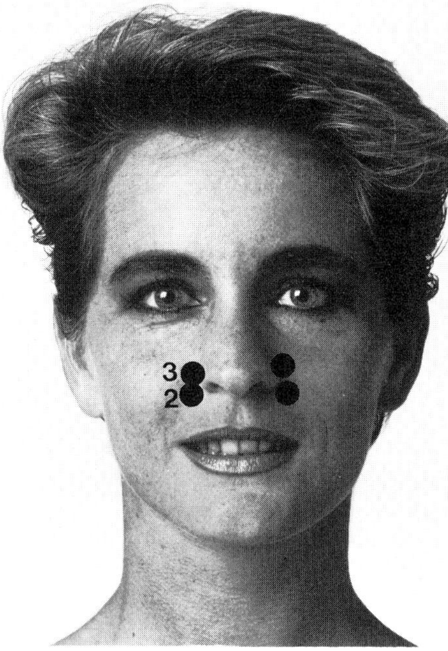


**Point 2** (S.I. 20) Left and right
Lies directly in the naso-labial groove on level with the nostrils.
**Point 3** (S.I. 19) Left and right
Located to the side of the nostrils, several millimeters next to the naso-labial fold.
**Point 4** (L. 7) Left and right
Located 2 fingerbreadths away from the wrist fold in the so-called radial groove.

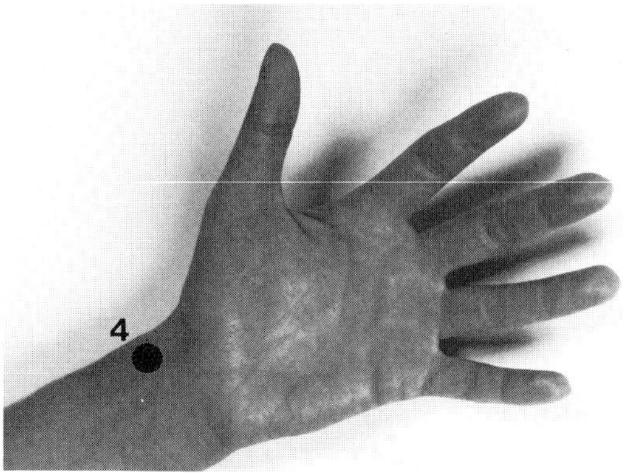

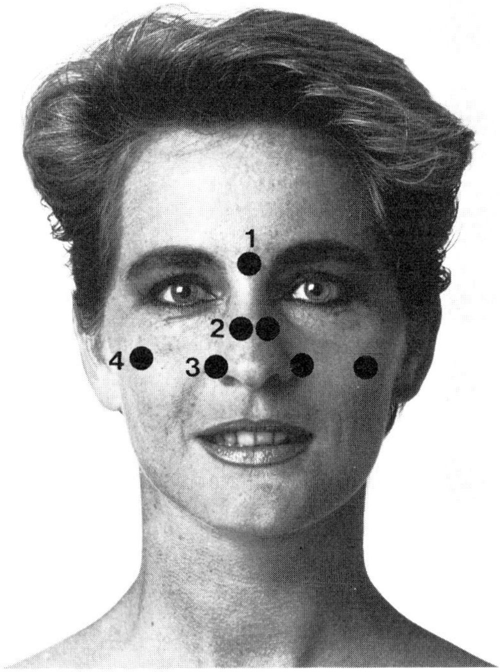


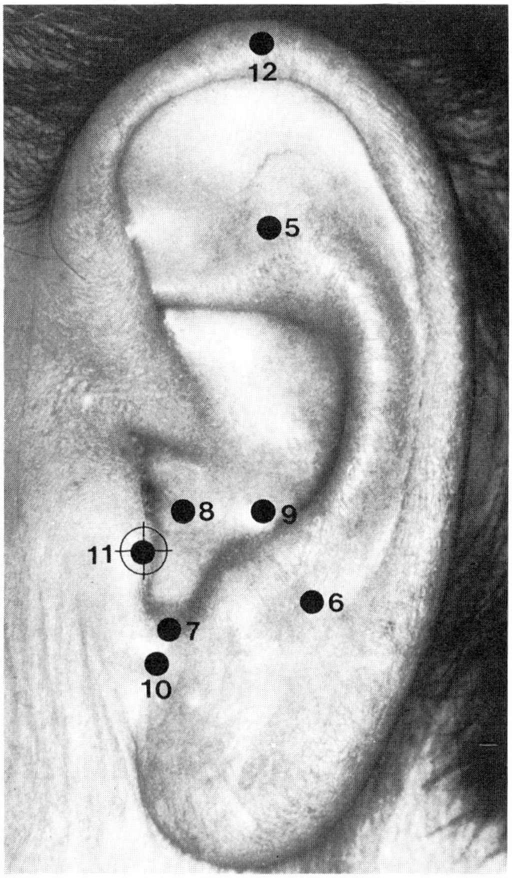


In addition to the above-mentioned points:

**Point 1**
(Yin trang)
Lies exactly on the midline between the eyebrows.

**Point 2**
(Cartilage points)
Situated to the left and the right of the midline of the bridge of the nose at the beginning of the nasal bone.

**Point 3**
(L.I. 20)
Lies directly in the naso-labial groove on level with the nostrils.

**Point 4**
(S.I. 18)
Situated on the cheek bone, on a vertical line descending from the outer corners of the eyes in a small hollow which can be felt there.

**Point 5:** Ear point
**Point 6:** Ear point
**Point 7:** Ear point
**Point 8:** Ear point
**Point 9:** Ear point
**Point 10:** Ear point
**Point 11:** Ear point
**Point 12:** Ear point

Acne, like any other skin disease, is associated with metabolic functioning as a whole. Deficient eliminatory processes must be impro-ved and a healthy, balanced diet adhered to. Pork and sugar are two items which should be eliminated altogether.
Begin by treating the points for activating the metabolism (see pp. 81 – 83) and the combination Energy Balancing II in daily alteration for ten days. Next treat the following special points for acne for 8 days. Finally employ the three combinations in daily alteration

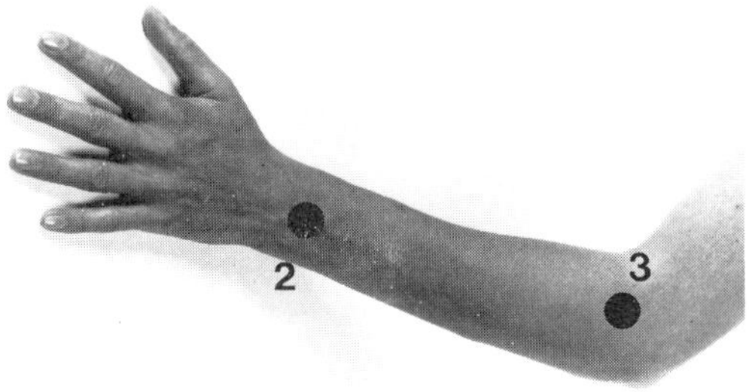


**Point 2** (T.H. 5)
Located approx. 2½ fingerbreadths above the wrist fold in the middle between the ulna and the radius.
**Point 3** (L.I. 11)
Located at the end of the upper elbow fold.

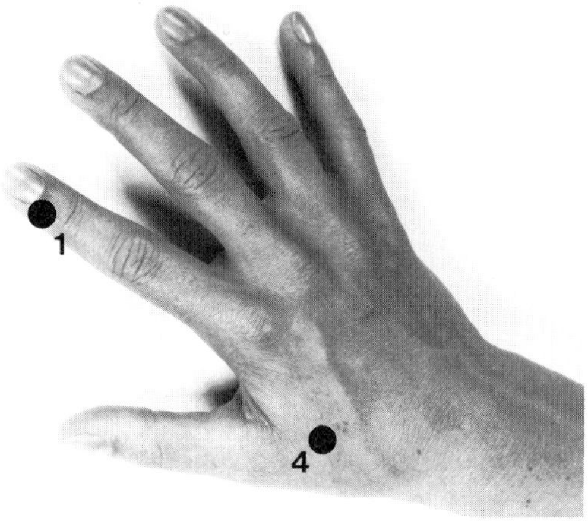


**Point 1**
(L.I. 1)
This point is located on medial surface of the distal phalanx of the index finger approx. 2 mm diagonally offset from the angle of the nailbed groove.
**Point 4**
(L.I. 4)
Located on the medial surface of the index finger in the angle formed by the thumb and the index finger.

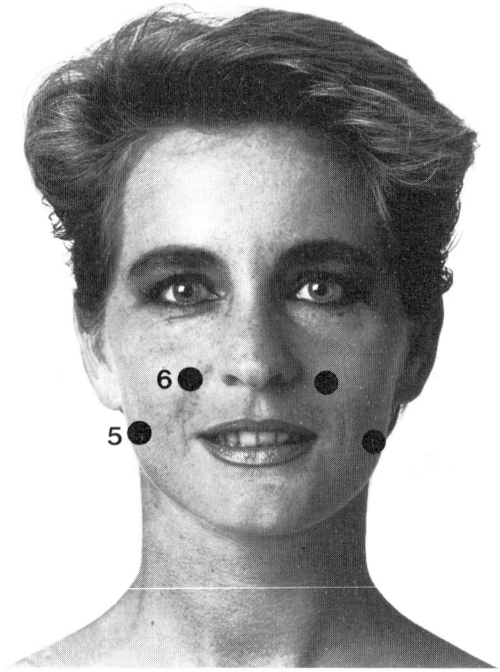


**Point 5** (Sp. 3)
Situated at the angle of the lower jaw.
**Point 6** (Sp. 6)
Located 1 fingerbreadth next to the nostril.

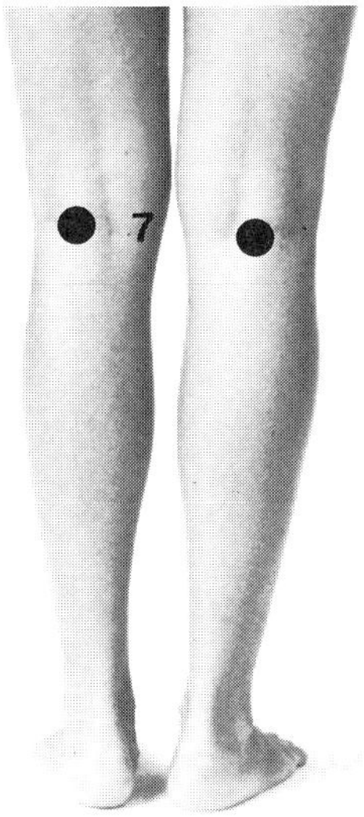


**Point 7**
(U.B. 54)
Located in the middle of the hollow of the knee.

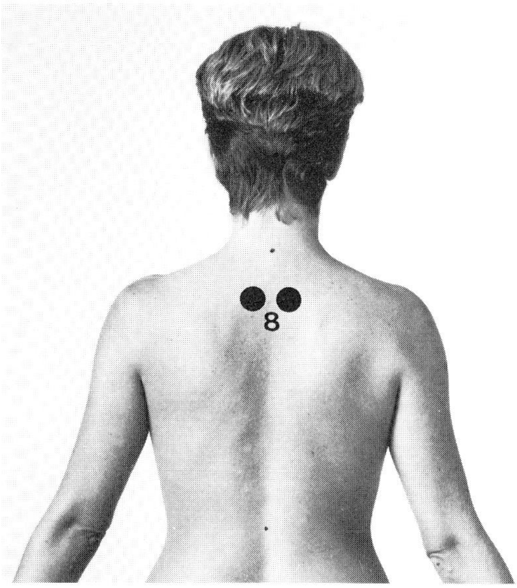


**Point 8**
(U.B. 13)
Located in the 3rd intercostal space, 2 finger-breadths away from the midline.

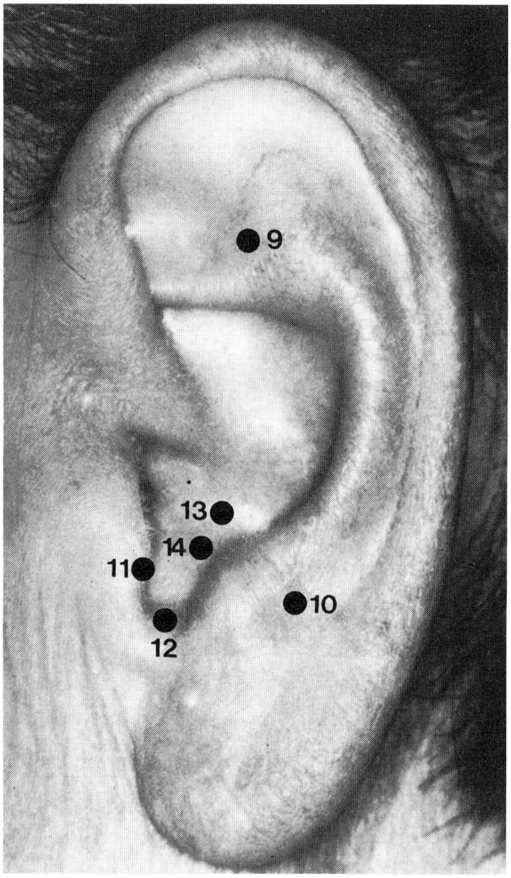


**Point 9:** Ear point
**Point 10:** Ear point
**Point 11:** Ear point
**Point 12:** Ear point
**Point 13:** Ear point
**Point 14:** Ear point

In cases of acne during puberty use the following points:

1st day: Lymph treatment with Energy Balancing I
2nd day: Control I
3rd day: Acne Combination
Continue in this manner.
Acne during puberty requires additional treatment with homöopathic or herbal medicines as indicated.

Intestinal functioning plays a particularly important part in acne, as do the metabolic and eliminatory processes. A healthy, balanced diet is therefore of paramount importance, as previously mentioned. A disturbed balance of the intestinal flora should be treated by an experienced physician or health practitioner. In cases of acne which are associated with constipation, include the points for constipation as specified here:

1. Treat the constipation points for 8 days.
2. Treat the metabolic points in daily alteration with the constipation points for 10 days.
3. Treat the points for constipation, metabolic functioning and acne and alternate daily.

# Heart Diseases

# Heart Segments

Persons suffering from heart disease should always seek the advice of an experienced physician or a licensed health practitioner and should not attempt to treat their complaints themselves. The acu-impulsor shows good results as an accompanying form of therapy, which is no wonder when one considers that harmonizing the flow of energy will contribute to the regeneration of any organ of the body.
On the other hand, there are a great number of complaints which supposedly have to do with the heart yet which are caused by other factors. In many instances of pain in the region of the heart, there are no relevant diagnostic findings so that the complaints are declared as being mere stress symptoms. There are, however, a number of other causes which may be responsible for heart complaints, such as abdominal distention, elevation of the diaphragm or spinal disorders. Lastly there are instances where stress does indeed cause such symptoms as stitches in the heart and cramping pain which may extend to the spine or down the left arm. All heart complaints must be thoroughly diagnosed before they can be treated with the acu-impulsor. When applied properly, this method has shown excellent results.

1. As a basic rule the Energy Balancing II combination is carried out as an initial measure which will improve the flow of the lymph from above and below via the chest and lung region. This combination will also strengthen the immune system.

2. The following points will have a general positive effect on the heart:

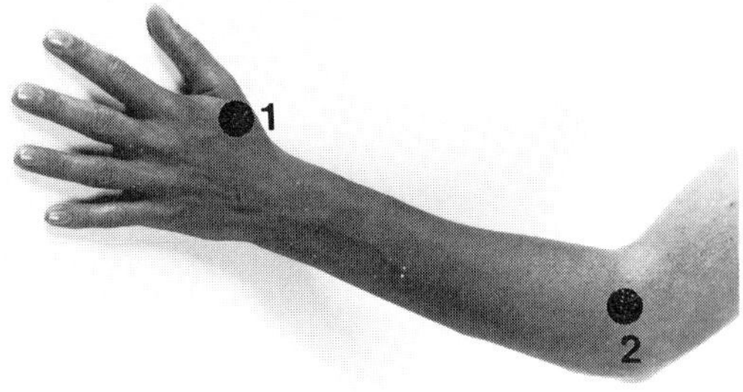


**Point 1**
(S.I. 4) Left and right
Located on the lateral surface of the index finger in the angle formed by the thumb and the index finger.

**Point 2**
(S.I. 11) Left and right
Located at the end of the upper elbow fold when the arm is slightly flexed.

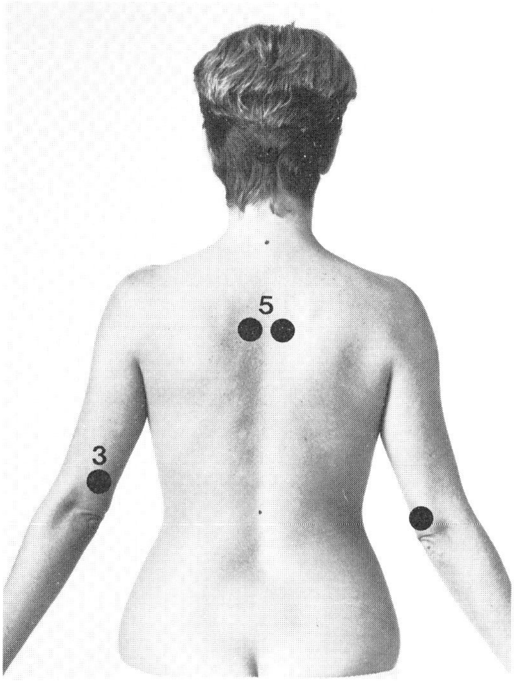


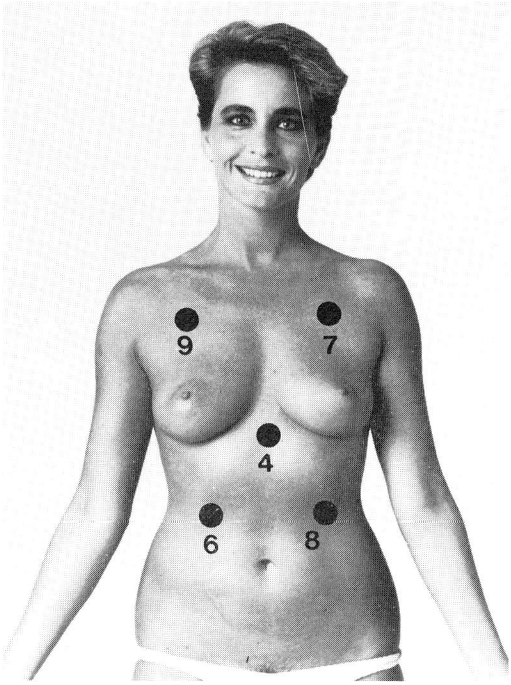


**Point 3**
(T.H. 10) Left and right
Located in a small hollow situated on the posterior surface of the extended arms.

**Point 4**
(C.V. 14)
Located on the midline of the body approx. 1 fingerbreadth below the tip of the xiphoid.

**Point 5**
(U.B. 15) Left and right
Located in the 5th intercostal space, 2 fingerbreadths offset from the midline.

In addition to these acupuncture points there are a number of zones which I discovered during the course of my work with EEA and Colorpuncture.

**Point 6**
(Right abdominal point)
Located in the upper right abdominal region, approx. 3 fingerbreadths away from the costal arch.

**Point 7**
(Left thoracic point)
Located in the upper left thoracic region, approx. 1 hand's breadth offset from the nipple. This point will be found to be painful on pressure.

**Point 8**
(Left abdominal point)
Located in the upper left abdominal region, approx. 3 fingerbreadths away from the costal arch.

**Point 9** (Right thoracic point)
Located in the upper right thoracic region, approx. 1 hand's breadth offset from the nipple. This point will be found to be painful on pressure.

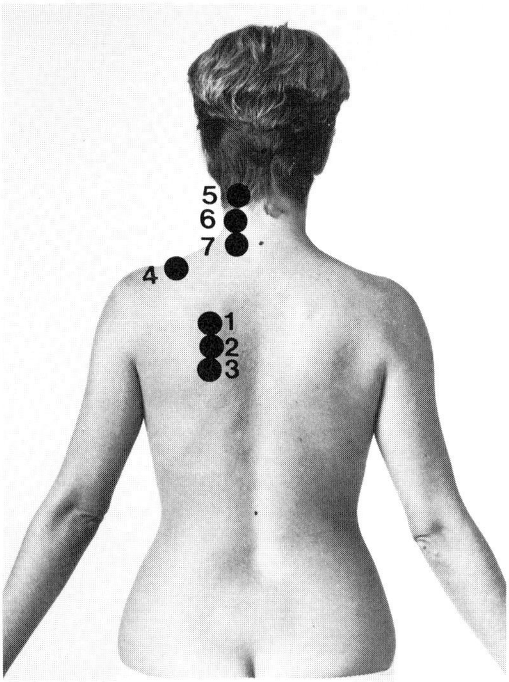


In all heart diseases the following segments on the back can be included in treatment. The points are all located on the left side.

**Points 1, 2 and 3**
Situated on the left margin of the shoulder blade.

**Point 4**
Situated directly on the shoulder, approx. 1 fingerbreadth laterally of the midpoint of the shoulder.

**Points 5, 6 and 7**
Located on the left side of the cervical spine, approx. 2 fingerbreadths away from the midline.

The points of this combination must be located by palpation. Each point specified is in fact a larger zone with a central point which is sensitive to touch.

# Ringing in the Ears

# Facial Pain

# Nasal Obstruction

# Suppression of Excessive Appetite

# Impotency

# Frigidity

The various kinds of noises some people experiences in their ears can be more than merely annoying when they persist for a longer period of time. While such noises do not cause any pain, they can indeed drive the individual to despair, particularly when all else around is peaceful and quiet.

Unfortunately, there are many cases which do not respond to treatment. Acupuncture, Colorpuncture and also acu-impulsor therapy have been able to achieve good results. While not all persons can be cured, it is possible to improve the complaints in many instances. In view of the fact that it has been possible to cure a considerable number of sufferer it is well worth trying acu-impulsor therapy. As in many other chronic complaints a great deal of patience is required. Other contributing factors such as lymphatic complaints of the sinuses or the ears must also be considered.

Therefore it is important to improve the flow of the lymph in the region of the head and also to improve the circulation in general.
The following points and zones should be treated daily, whereby Energy Balancing II is to be carried out in the morning (repeat twice) and the specific points for ringing in the ears are treated in the evening.
Once again, I would like to remind you that the successful treatment of these unpleasant symptoms requires a considerable amount of patience.

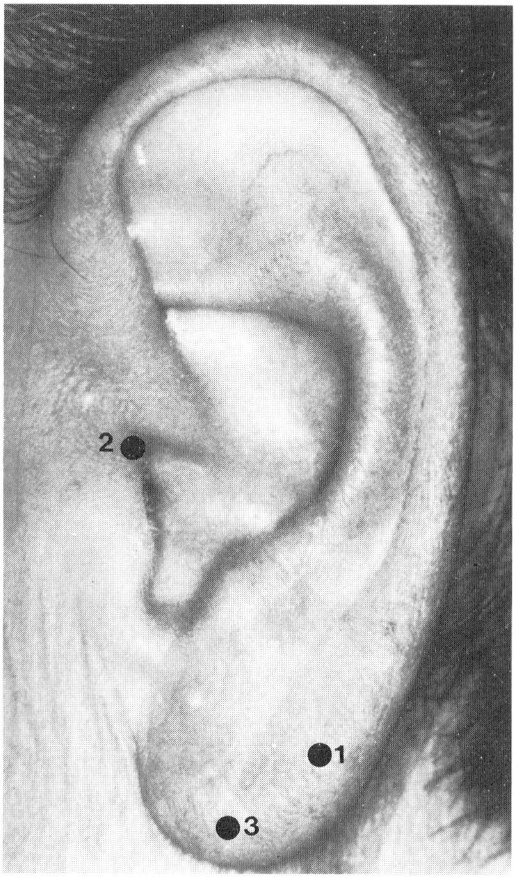


**Point 1:** Ear point
**Point 2:** Ear point
**Point 3:** Ear point

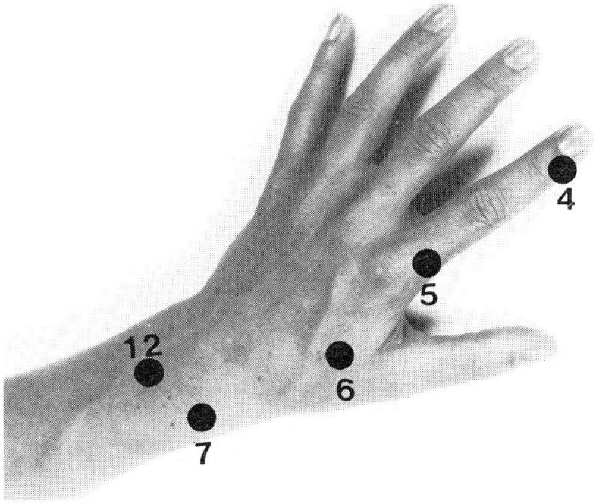


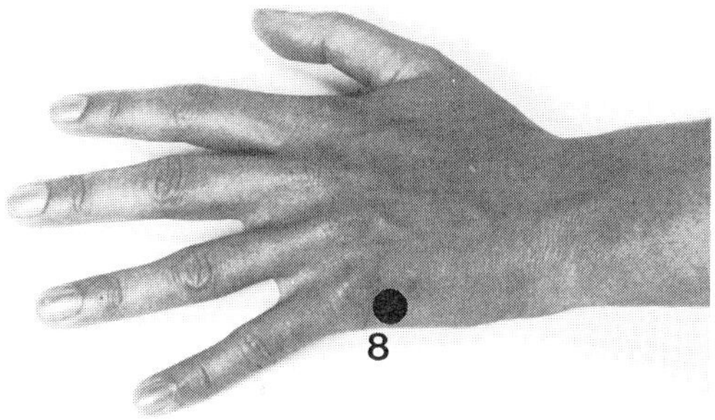


**Point 4**
(L.I. 1) Left and right
Located on the medial side of the distal phalanx of the index finger approx. 2 mm diagonally offset from the angle of the nailbed groove.

**Point 5**
(L.I. 2) Left and right
Located on the medial side approx. ½ fingerbreadth offset from the basal joint of the index finger.

**Point 6**
(L.I. 4) Left and right
Located on the medial side of the index finger in the angle formed by the thumb and the index finger.

**Point 7**
(L.I. 6)
Situated approx. 3 fingerbreadths above the wrist fold in a small hollow which can be felt there.

**Point 12**
(T.H. 5) Left and right
Located approx. 2½ fingerbreadths above the wrist fold in the middle between ulna and radius.

**Point 8**
(S.I. 3) Left and right
Located at the end of a fold which is formed above the basal joint of the small finger by making a fist.

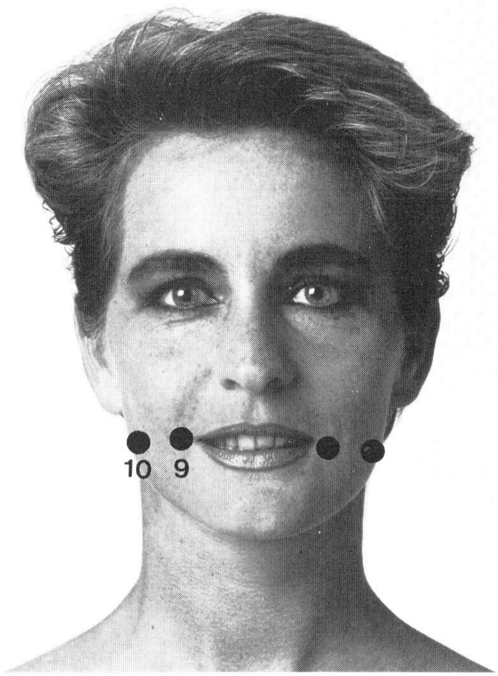


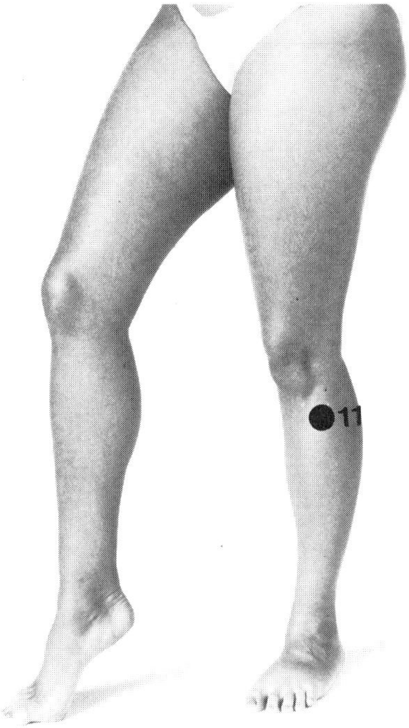


**Point 9**

(St. 7) Left and right

Located approx. ½ fingerbreadth offset from the corner of the mouth.

**Point 10**

(St. 3) Left and right

Located at the lower angle of the jaw.

**Point 11**

(St. 36) Left and right

This point is located on the anterior, medial surface of the lower leg, 3 fingerbreadths below the knee, in the middle of the shin bone. This point can also be found by placing the palm of the hand on the kneecap, in which case the tip of the middle finger will indicate the position of the point.

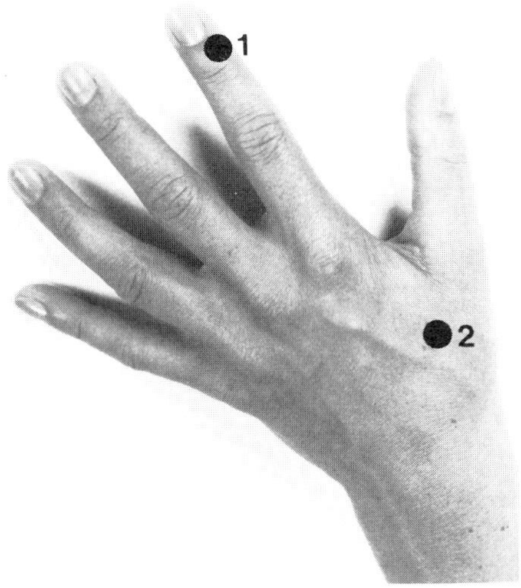


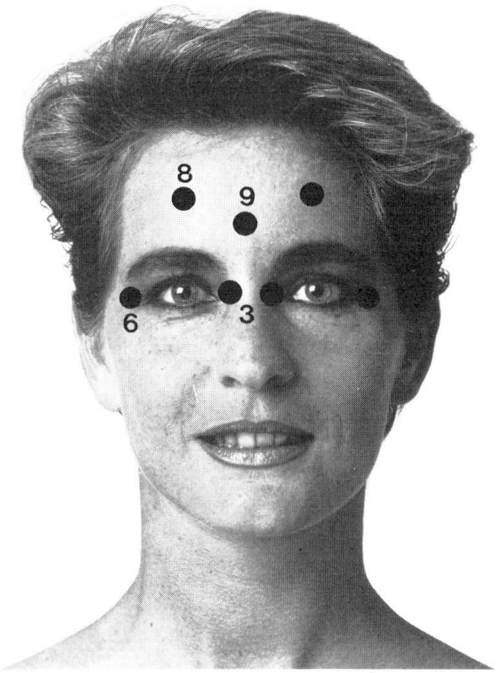


**Point 1**
(L.I. 1) Left and right
Located on the distal phalanx of the index finger, 2 mm diagonally offset from the medial angle of the nailbed groove.

**Point 2**
(L.I. 4) Left and right
Located on the medial surface of the index finger, in the angle formed by the thumb and the index finger.

**Point 3**
(U.B. 1) Left and right
Located at the inner upper angle of the orbita.

**Point 6**
(G.B. 1) Left and right
Located in the angle formed by the external margin of the eyebrow arch and the cheek bone.

**Point 8**
(Hypothalamus point)
Located on a line extending vertically from the center of the eye, in the middle of the forehead.

**Point 9**
(Limbic system)
The first point is located 2 fingerbreadths above the point situated exactly between the eyebrows. This point must always be determined by palpation and should only be treated if it is found to be painful.

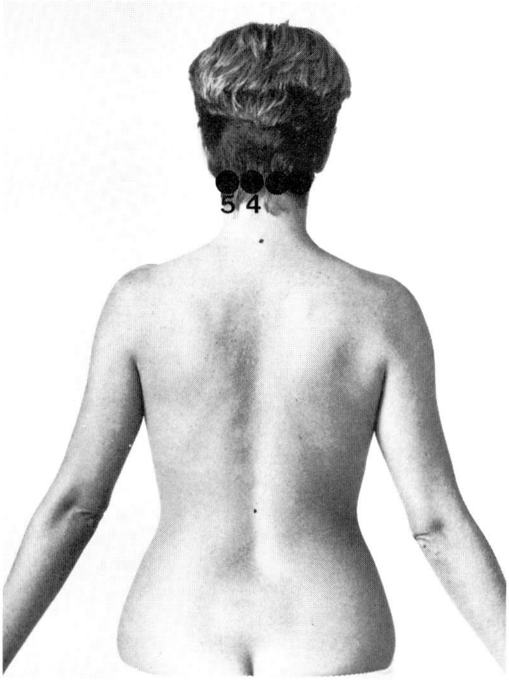


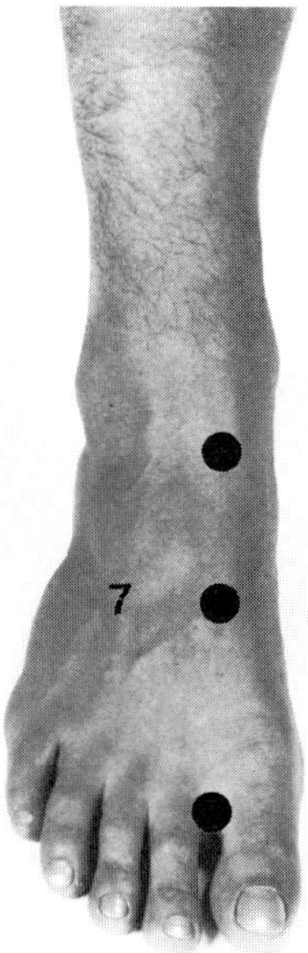


**Point 4**

(U.B. 10) Left and right

Located approx. 1 fingerbreadth below the squamous part of the occipital bone and 1½ fingerbreadths offset from the midline of the body. This point will be found to be painful on touch.

**Point 5**

(G.B. 20) Left and right

Located in a hollow approx. 3 fingerbreadths away from the midline and 1 fingerbreadth beneath the medial section of the squamous part of the occipital bone.

**Point 7**

(Lymph points on the foot) Left and right

These lymph points are actually larger zones, whereby only their midpoints are treated. The first midpoint is situated on the upper margin of the web between the 1st and 2nd toe. The 2nd is located at the middle of the foot on a line extending from the first point along the back of the foot. The third point is located in the fold of the ankle joint.

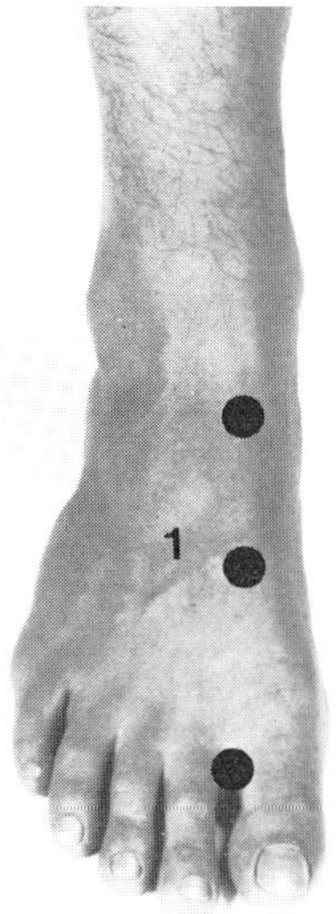


**Point 1**
(Lymph points on the foot) Left and right
These lymph points are actually larger zones, whereby only their midpoints are treated. The first midpoint is situated on the upper margin of the web between the 1st and 2nd toe. The 2nd is located at the middle of the foot on a line extending from the first point along the back of the foot. The third point is located in the fold of the ankle joint.

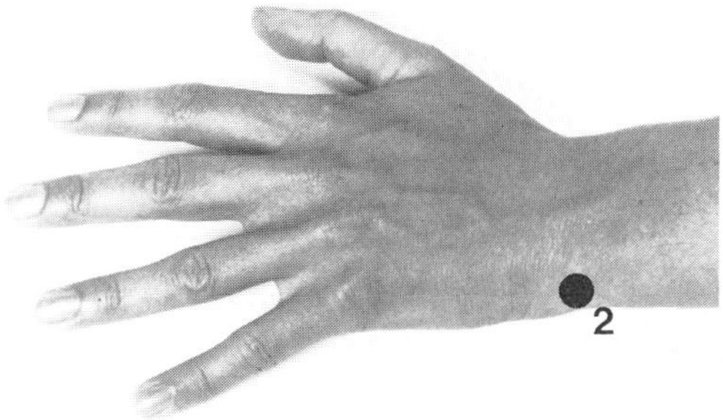


**Point 2** (S.I. 4) Left and right
Located on the lateral surface of the hand where a small gap of the joint can be felt.

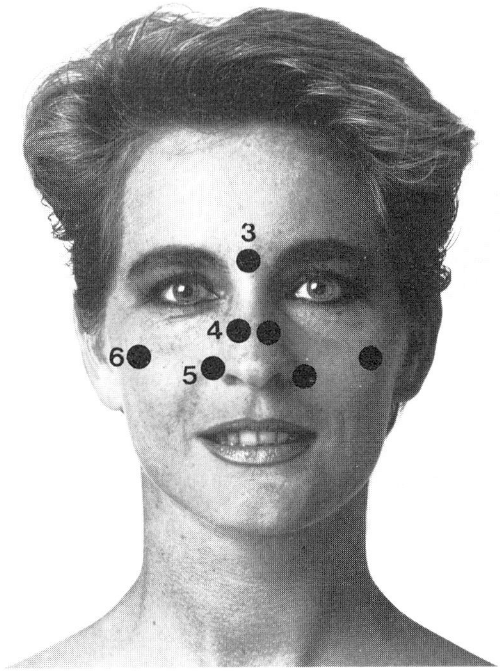


**Point 3**
(Yin trang)
This point is located exactly on the midline between the eyebrows.

**Point 4**
(Cartilage point)
Located on the bridge of the nose to the right and the left of the midline, next to the nasal bone.

**Point 5**
(L.I. 20) Left and right
Located on both sides of the nostrils, several millimeters next to the naso-labial groove.

**Point 6**
(S.I.18) Left and right
Located on the cheek bone in a small hollow on vertical line beginning at the external angle of the eye.

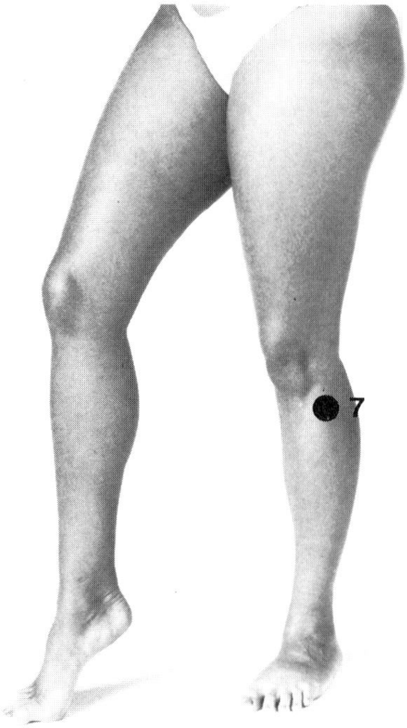


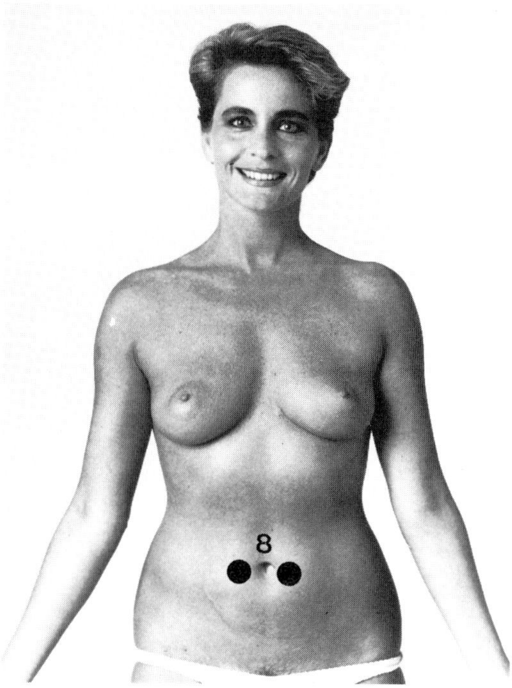


**Point 7**

(St. 36) Left and right

This point is located on the anterior, medial surface of the lower leg, 3 fingerbreadths below the knee, in the middle of the shin bone. This point can also be found by placing the palm of the hand on the kneecap, in which case the tip of the middle finger will indicate the position of the point.

**Point 8**

(St. 25) Left and right

Located 2 fingerbreadths away from the center of the navel.

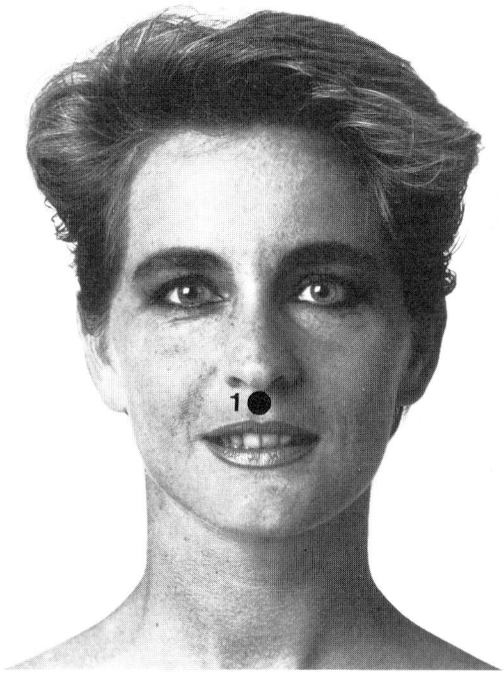


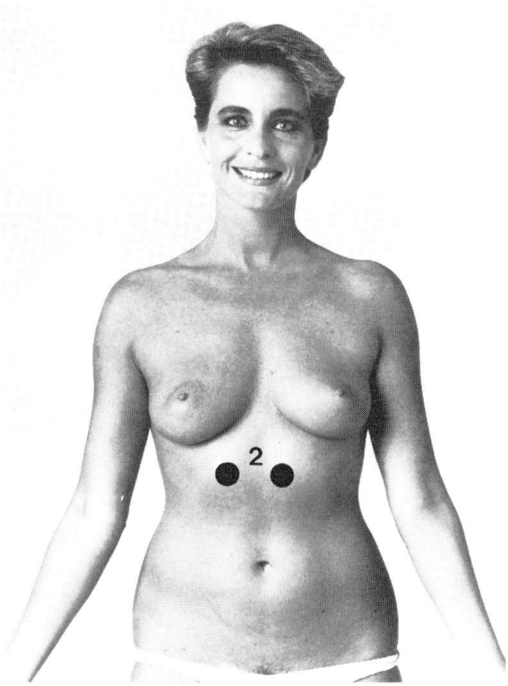


**Point 1**
(G.V. 26)
Located on the upper lip, directly under the nose.

**Point 2**
(St. 19) Left and right
Situated directly on the costal arch, 2 fingerbreadths next to the midline of the body.

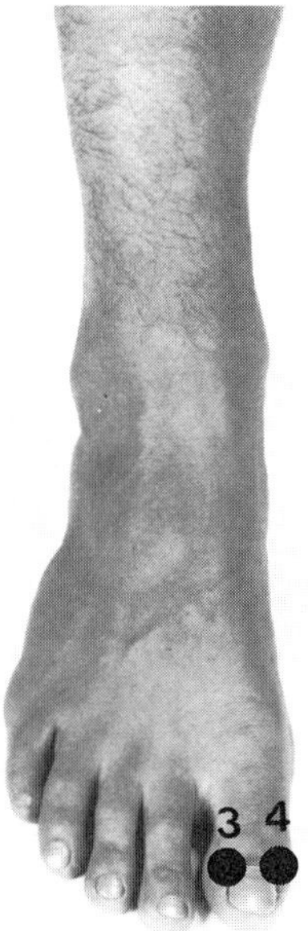


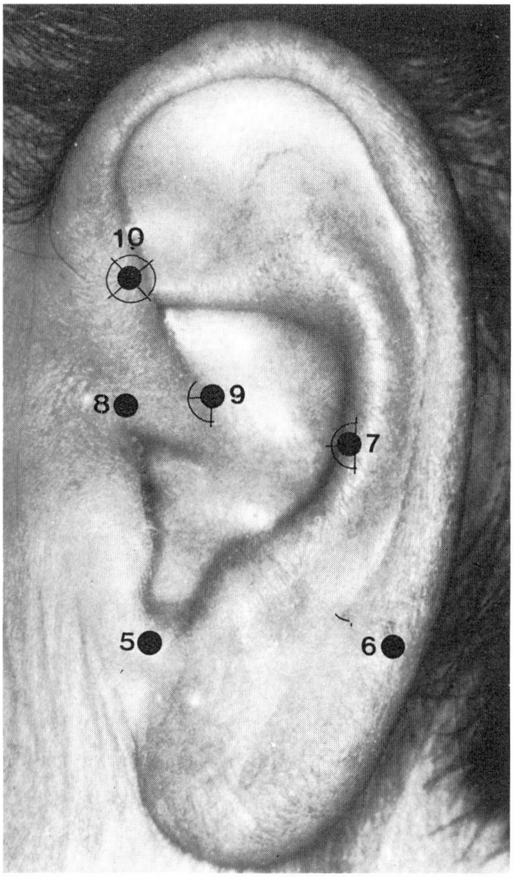


**Point 3**

(Liv. 3) Left and right

Located on the lateral side of the big toe, 2 mm diagonally offset from the angle of the nailbed groove.

**Point 4**

(P. 1) Left and right

Located on the distal phalanx of the big toe, on the medial side, approx. 2 mm offset from the angle of the nailbed groove.

**Point 5:** Ear point
**Point 6:** Ear point
**Point 7** Ear point
**Point 8:** Ear point
**Point 9:** Ear point
**Point 10:** Ear point

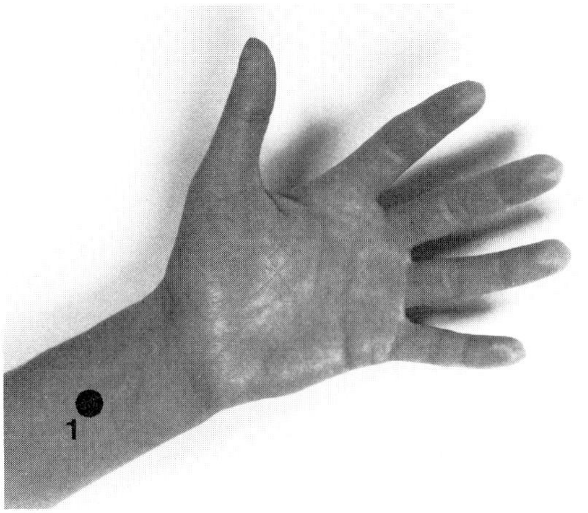


**Point 1**
(C. 6) Left and right
Located approx. 3 fingerbreadths above the first wrist fold on the medial surface of the forearm in the middle.

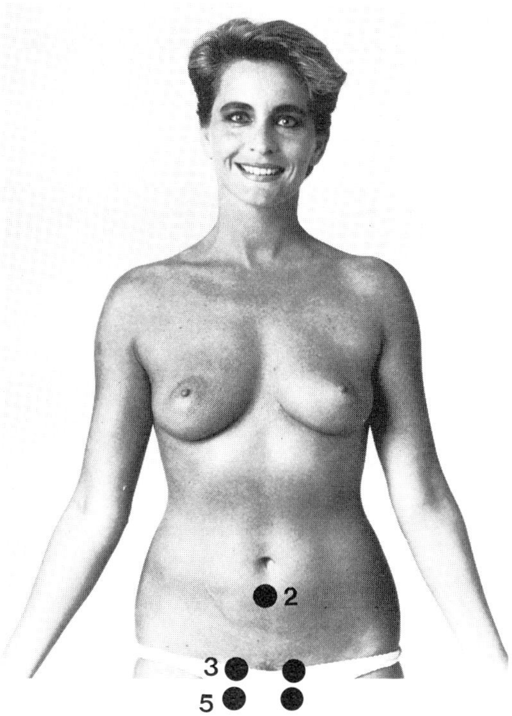


**Point 2**
(C.V. 6)
Located on the midline of the body approx. 2 fingerbreadths below the navel.

**Point 3**
(St. 30) Left and right
Located on the lower margin of the pubic bone, 2 fingerbreadths away from the midline of the body.

**Point 5**
(K. 11) Left and right
Located on the upper margin of the pubic bone, 2 fingerbreadths away from the midline of the body.

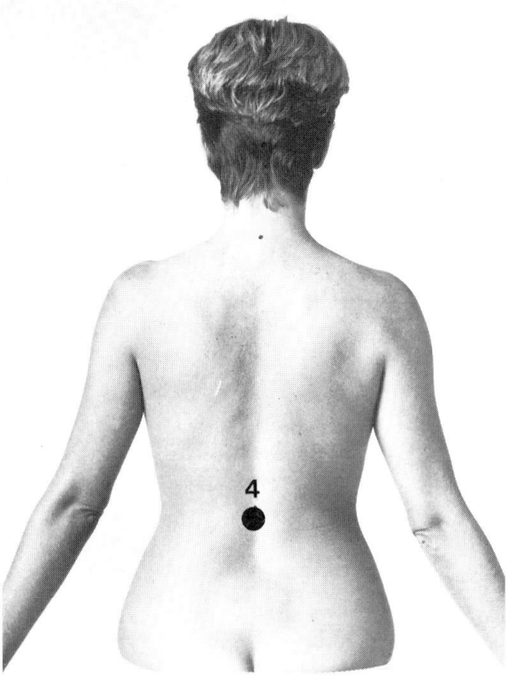


**Point 4**
(G.V. 4)
Situated on the spinal process of the 2 lumbar vertebra.

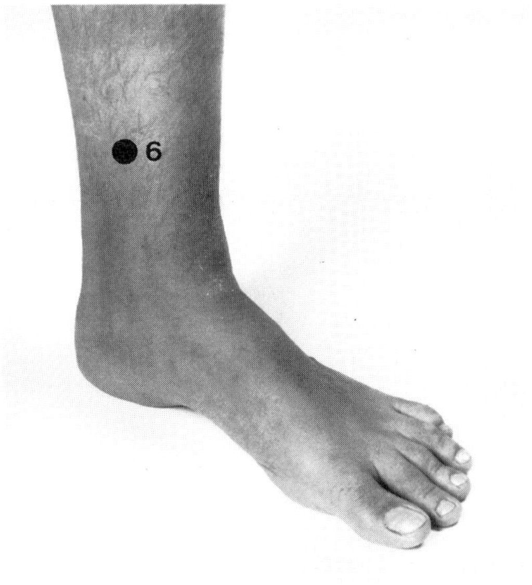


**Point 6**
(P. 6) Left and right
Located on the medial surface of the ankle, about 4 fingerbreadths above the ankle bone.

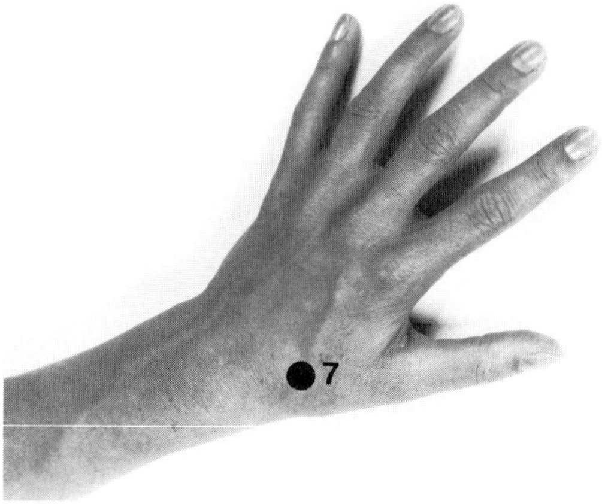


**Point 7** (S.I. 5) Left and right
Located on the medial side of the wrist, at the upper end of a small hollow which is formed when the thumb is extended.

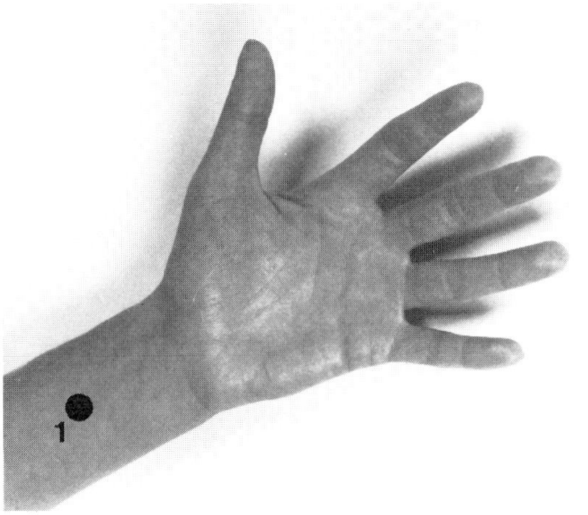


**Point 1**
(C. 6) Left and right
Located approx. 3 fingerbreadths above the first fold of the wrist on the medial surface of the forearm in the middle.

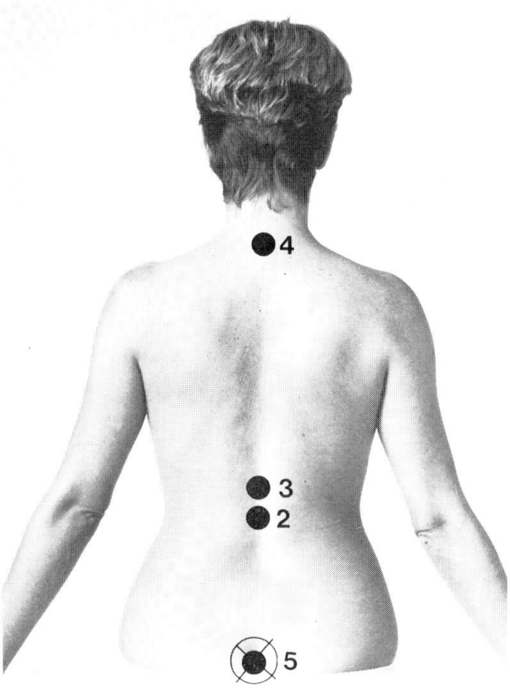


**Point 2**
(G.V. 4)
Located on the spinal process of the 2nd lumbar vertebra.

**Point 3**
(G.V. 5)
Located on the spinal process of the 1st lumbar vertebra.

**Point 4**
(G.V. 13)
Situated directly on the tip of the spinal process of the 7th cervical vertebra.

**Point 5**
(G.V. 1)
Located on the midline of the body at the lower end of the coccyx.

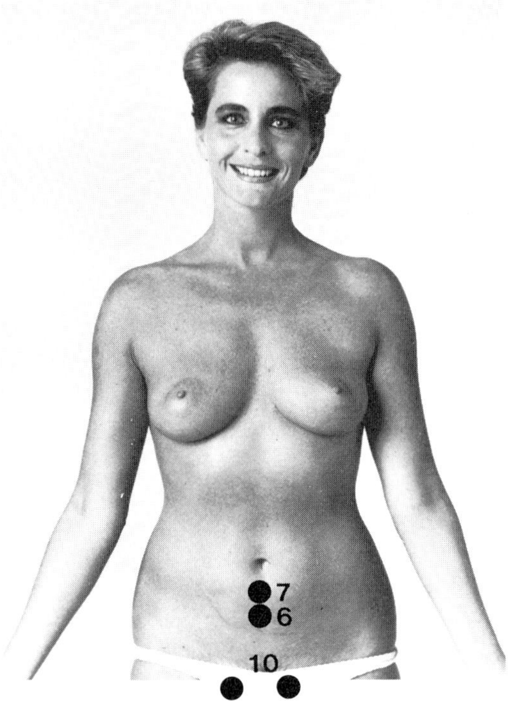


**Point 6**
(C.V. 5)
This point is located on the lower margin of the first third of the line connecting the pubic bone and the navel.

**Point 7**
(C.V. 6)
Located 2 fingerbreadths below the navel on the midline of the body.

**Point 10**
(K. 11) Left and right
Located on the upper margin of the pubic bone, 2 fingerbreadths offset from the midline of the body.

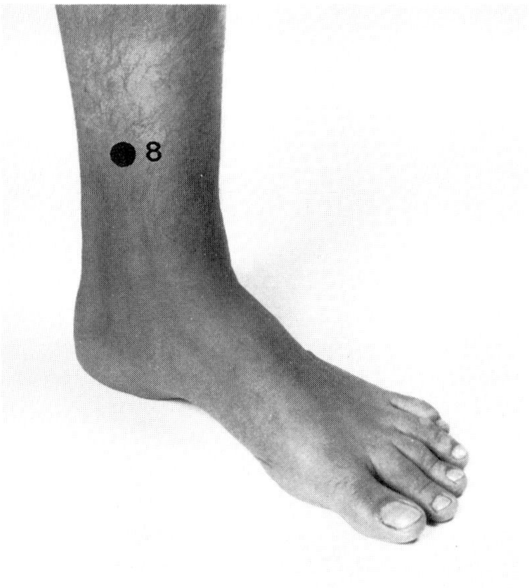


**Point 8**
(P. 6) Left and right
Situated on the medial surface of the ankle, approx. 4 fingerbreadths above the ankle-bone.

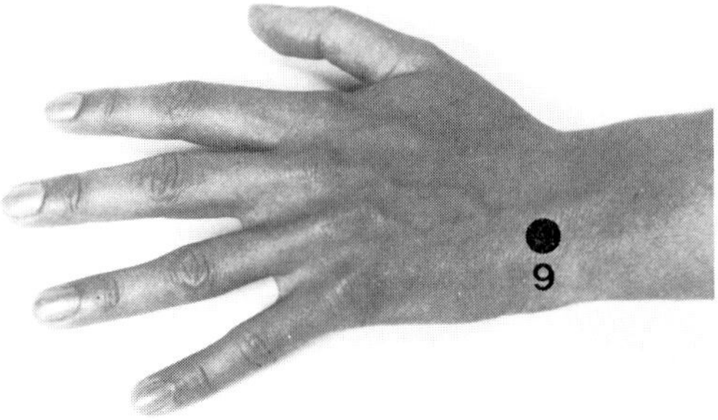


**Point 9**
(T.H. 4) Left and right
Located on the wrist fold on the back of the hand, between the ring finger and the small finger.

# Conclusion

I wrote this book in the sincere conviction that the awareness of man's inherent physical and psychological balance is steadily increasing and that therefore effective self-treatment – which must always be carried out under the supervision of an experienced practitioner – is becoming an indispensable component in the preservation and restoration of health. More and more people are realizing the necessity to take responsibility for their health.

Our knowledge of man's energetic structure and the fact that reaction cannot take place without information makes acu-impulsor therapy one of the foremost self-help methods.

I hope that this book will be read by a large number of people. I believe it could make a considerable contribution toward the safe and effective treatment of a number of diseases caused by the detrimental effects of modern civilization and those disorders so often done away with as being merely "minor complaints". It is particularly in the field of prophylaxis that the acu-impulsor is capable of achieving outstanding results. It is always preferable to improve one's level of health than to allow it to deteriorate by doing nothing at all. Remember, the treatment of manifest disease and the restoration to a state of health will always require more time and effort than that involved by prophylactic measures.